In the year 2100, death from aging-associated disease will seem as unusual as death due to infection now is in affluent industrialized countries.

- Professor Michael R. Rose,
University of California, Irvine

LIVE FOREVER MANUAL

101 Practical Tips on How to Live Forever

By Adrian Cull

For more information and the latest life extension news, visit the website: https://liveforever.club

In memory of loved ones who have died whilst writing this book, including my Grandma, who had a good innings at 93, and my dearest friend Scott, who at 47 did not.

With thanks to my partner, Ann, whose support has allowed me to spend too much time at my desk researching and writing, and who's realism has highlighted to me how hard it is to convince people that, yes, I really mean we may be able to live forever.

TABLE OF CONTENTS

TABLE OF CONTENTS

TABLE OF CONTENTS

Introduction

> The day before something is truly a breakthrough, it's a crazy idea.
> - Peter Diamandis

The thought of living forever may sound like a doubly crazy idea – crazy to want to live longer when most people accept their fate by the time they reach their old age, and secondly, crazy that it could ever be possible, let alone within our lifetime.

So, let me make this important point first and foremost. Nobody's goal is to live forever in a wheelchair, in decrepitude, or in pain. As I will try my best to demonstrate in this book, scientists already working in the field of ageing research and life extension see no boundary between the techniques required to cure age-related disease (for example, to remove artery plaques that cause heart attacks and strokes) and the procedures that slow ageing itself. Nor do they see any boundaries between the methods that reduce ageing and those that reverse it – they all form the same giant mountain of a challenge. We are still at the very bottom of it, but we can see the top and already have a plan to get us to base camp. As we start our journey, we will discover more about the mountain's structure and we'll learn new techniques to scale it and to reach its peak. By the time we arrive at the top no-one will be dying of diseases that are triggered by the accumulated damage of ageing. People will be able to live in the bodies of their twenties with no risk of physical or mental deterioration, able to fully enjoy the experience of life for as long as they choose. Conventional wisdom says that this is impossible, and the general scientific community has barely even woken up to the idea. However, in my opinion this belief comes from a lack of awareness of recent advances in our knowledge of how the body ages, combined with the very human inability to see beyond current assumptions and to radically change one's mindset.

These types of paradigm shifts have happened in the past. For example the Copernican model, which put the sun at the centre of the solar system instead of the Earth, faced harsh when it was first proposed. This despite the fact that the supporters of the incumbent model were having to come up with more and more outlandish explanations of planetary movements to support their own views.

More recently, the impossibility of powered flight was the accepted view until very shortly before it happened. In 1896, Lord Kelvin, who discovered the second law of thermodynamics, said he had "not the smallest molecule of faith in aerial navigation other than ballooning." In December 1901, the engineer-in-chief of the US Navy, Rear Admiral George W. Melville, argued against "aerial navigation" based on themes including nature knows best, its physical impossibility and the wasteful use of resources – themes which are also used as arguments against curing ageing today. Two years later, in October 1903, the New York Times suggested powered flight would not be achieved within a million years and Simon Newcomb, President of the American Astronomical Society - so someone who knew a thing or two about physics - claimed that "aerial flight is one the great class of problem with which man can never cope." That was just two months before the Wright brothers made the first sustained flight of a powered, heavier-than-air aircraft.

So it is no surprise that established thinking is also slow to change in the area of ageing. Today some scientists are willing to accept that life expectancy could increase, with the people living, on average, to 100, but they believe that anything beyond that is an impossibility. Well, they've been saying that for a long time. In 1928, Louis Israel Dublin, a previous president of the American Statistical Association, wrote a report on the economics of world health that predicted a limit of sixty-five years for life expectancy. Unfortunately for Dublin, this limit had already been surpassed in New Zealand and is currently about 30% longer in most high-income countries.

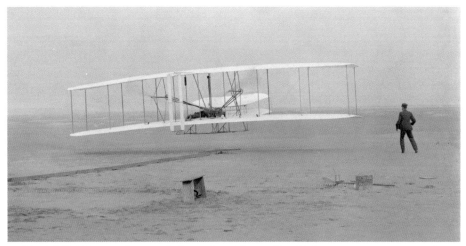

"Aerial flight is one the great class of problem with which man can never cope." - American Astronomical Society, 1903. Two months before the first powered flight.

As the first treatments arrive to chip away at the damage of ageing the naysayers will still be the ones heard the loudest, claiming it is all an impossible dream. And I appreciate the difficulty of foreseeing significant change: even the Wright brothers themselves, after having made their first diminutive flight, could not have imagined the aero industry that exists today.

I hope that by writing this book, I will free you from the despondency caused by the slow pace of medical improvements in the last century and open your eyes to the possibilities to come in the next few decades.

PART ONE – THE COMING LIFE EXTENSION REVOLUTION

The first half of this book introduces the science, ethics and technology of life extension, to provide you with some background to a movement that is bigger than most people realise. I wouldn't go as far as to call it an underground movement, but given the derision that researchers have faced for decades, many academics are careful when speaking about the possible impacts of scientific advances. It is only recently that advocates have emerged, who are willing to say that ageing and death are bad and should be stopped.

In the first chapter, *Can you really live forever* I explain that, even accepting how long people have incorrectly thought we were on the verge of biological immortality, there are prominent and respected people who believe we really can get there. I also highlight some animals that show we have the potential to live significantly longer.

But even if we can, you may have concerns about whether we should. So, in *Should we?* I will address these arguments, such as whether it is natural and how would we live without death.

If, after that chapter, I've managed to persuade you that seeking to extend life is a worthwhile endeavour, you may still worry about the consequences of its success. Will only the rich live forever? Will people currently in power (as leaders of companies and countries) be in power indefinitely? How will the planet cope? I discuss all of these concerns in *But, what if?*

Then I start to dig a little deeper. The *What is ageing?* chapter examines the underlying causes of ageing – physical markers that explain why people who have lived for the same number of years may have different biological ages.

Biological detail is examined further in *Curing ageing*, where each of the seven fundamental mechanisms that cause age-related damage to the body are discussed along with the current thinking on how each and every one of them can be fixed.

Life extension research uses terms such as healthspan, longevity, and escape velocity; so, I explain these in *Life extension glossary* I also illustrate how they all relate together on a chart showing chronological versus biological age.

Given the current state of healthcare, where cancer is often terminal, and where most diseases have no known cure (only treatments to alleviate the symptoms), I realise it is hard to believe this could all be eradicated in the near future. I'm not saying it will, but in the *Outrunning death* chapter I explain how each medical advancement will buy you more time until the next one appears.

Just how fast do these advances have to come? Is it reasonable to assume we'll see a deluge of new discoveries and treatments? In *Exponential improvements in technology* I explain why this is far more likely than you might think, and I give a retrospective on Moore's Law and also look forwards to the technological singularity.

Then in *Advances in medical technology* I provide examples of have technological improvements are rapidly changing the face of medicine.

So that you don't have to just take my word for it, in the *Putting their money where their mouth is* chapter I reveal the people, companies, and investment funds all putting significant time and money into the life extension industry. It is one thing to hope and believe that something will happen, and another to believe it earnestly enough to spend millions of dollars on it.

Before you start spending your hard-earned money on anti-ageing treatments, make sure you read *Fountains of youth*, where I list some of the not-so-proven, and sometimes downright dangerous, remedies that you are likely to come across.

PART TWO - THE TIPS

The second part of this book offers 101 practical tips that can start you on the race to outrun death. Each has been researched and checked, to the best of my ability, against the latest and most comprehensive scientific research.

Newspapers love to shout about trials that have unconventional or extreme results and are happy to use them for a snappy headline one day and to forget about it the next, so they should always be taken with a pinch of salt. Consider how many people were involved in the trial. If it was only a handful, then remember that random variation will generate any result you want, if you run the experiment enough times. Was the experiment even done on people? Many, many biological impacts on cells in other animals do not have similar results in humans. What exactly was the benefit? "Super pill reduces heart attacks by 50%" makes a great clickbait headline, but it is significantly less attractive if the research details show a massive increase in mortality from other causes.

Use the tips as a handy reference to guide your lifestyle choices. Read them all or just dip in when looking for suggestions on a particular topic. As you will discover from reading part 1 of this book, the plan is to live long enough to live forever, and every day counts. Applying the tips that increase your life expectancy will improve your chances of benefiting from the ageing prevention therapies that are just around the corner, and which will lead to even greater life extension.

To misquote Lao Tzu: "A life of a thousand years begins with a single step."

Reading this manual is your first step.

Can we really live forever?

But there is nothing in biology yet found that indicates the inevitability of death. This suggests to me that it is not at all inevitable, and that it is only a matter of time before the biologists discover what it is that is causing us the trouble and that that terrible universal disease or temporariness of the human's body will be cured.
- Nobel Prize winning physicist Richard Phillips Feynman

Around the corner for millennia

People have been prophesising the arrival of immortality for thousands of years, though until recently, this has been wishful thinking rather than based on scientific prediction. The concept of eternal youth has always been around and can be found as far back as in early mythology and ancient religions. Although, for mere mortals, eternal life was something that was generally only attainable after death, with the notion of a soul's living forever rather than the human body surviving in perpetuity.

In the 5th century BCE, Herodotus wrote about the concept of a fountain of youth, that provided Macrobians with their exceptional longevity, and in the 3rd century BCE, there were legends of Alexander the Great crossing the Land of Darkness to find the spring of the water of life. This idea was not only found in the western world. In 219 BCE, Qin Shi Huang, founder of the Qin dynasty, sent his court sorcerer to search for Penglai Mountain, fabled to be home of immortals who held the elixir of life.

In art, the famous 1546 painting by Lucas Cranach the Elder shows elderly people being carried and aided to a pool where their wrinkled skin and tired expressions are rejuvenated, ready to enjoy youthful life again.

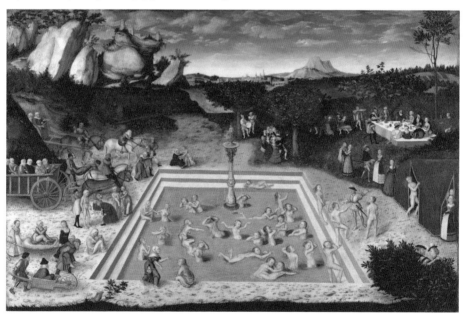

The Fountain of Youth - Lucas Cranach the Elder

Even esteemed scientists such as Isaac Newton (1642 - 1726) believed immortality was possible. As well as formulating the laws of motion and gravity he was also an alchemist (alchemy was the precursor to chemistry). He had a recipe for a Philosopher's Stone that would "transform lead into gold, but also help humans achieve immortality". Of course, he lived two centuries before even the basic germ theory of disease was accepted, so was oblivious to the complications of the cellular mechanisms of ageing, of which we now have a better understanding of.

Respected people think we can

Fortunately, as our knowledge has increased, the possibility of preventing ageing has become a crackable problem rather than a futile endeavour. That's not to say it will be easy, rather that now it is becoming increasingly clear what it will take to achieve.

A leading proponent of life extension is Ray Kurzweil. He invented the first commercial text-to-speech synthesizer and was awarded the National Medal of Technology and Innovation by President Clinton ,to go with his twenty-one honorary doctorates. In 2012, he became Google's director of engineering - this is a person worth listening too. He has used his knowledge of technology to make predictions, not only of what might happen but also how far off in the future it might occur. He has also been reasonably accurate at forecasting when computers would beat the best human chess players, the growth of the internet and the use of portable computers. So, when Ray looks into the future and predicts that by 2028, life expectancy will be increasing faster than we're living (see escape velocity in What Is Life Extension?) then he's got to be taken seriously. Even if he's wrong about the exact year it may be close enough to aim for.

Another presidential award recipient (2008 National Medal of Science) is Craig Venter. In 1984, he joined the National Institutes of Health and controversially attempted to patent some genes used in the brain. Continuing his entrepreneurial pursuits he formed Celera Genomics to commercialise genomic information, using shotgun sequencing to read the human genome for significantly less money than the Human Genome Project. He was the first person to have his complete DNA sequenced. 2010 saw Venter's team of scientists create the first synthetic life using manufactured DNA. Venter's latest venture is Human Longevity Inc., formed in 2013, a company which has raised $300m to end ageing through genomics and cell therapy.

Historically, academia has focussed on tackling individual diseases, and has shunned research into the underlying causes of ageing for fear of appearing as a modern Dr Victor Frankenstein. Fortunately, the tide is turning as more scientists realise that many diseases share common origins, which are often the same as, or eventually go on to cause, runaway ageing.

Harvard Medical School's Paul F. Glenn Center for the Biology of Ageing aims to slow ageing and to extend the healthy years of human life. Some of its recent research has successfully reversed the ageing of blood vessels in animals and David Sinclair, one of its co-directors, has developed a drug that is able to "reverse DNA damage and turn elderly mice into energetic young ones". Human trials are planned.

The Yale Center for Research on Ageing (Y-Age) focusses on translating the basic biology of ageing into treatments to promote healthy ageing and to combat common age-related diseases. It has recently doubled the number of compounds known to extend lifespan in yeast and one of its goals is to rejuvenate cells that have already reached old age – an essential part of living longer, younger.

In the UK, University College London's Institute of Healthy Ageing studies the biology of ageing and aims to protect against the diseases of old age. Recent research has shown that normal biological processes which are useful early on in life, continue to 'run-on' pointlessly in later life, causing age-related diseases. This discovery makes these possible targets for future therapies.

Newcastle University's Institute for Ageing is working on all aspects of ageing including medical, biological and cellular, with a vision of living better for longer. Thus this is an important point – it would be hard to find anyone who thought living longer would be of great benefit if we continued to age, becoming more and more decrepit and reliant on others. That is not the plan.

With a young mind and body

Geriatric medicine is concerned with treating the symptoms of age-related diseases rather than the disease of ageing itself. This does result in modestly longer lives, but at the expense of spending more time in poor health and decrepitude. That is not a desirable prospect when the length of lives may be radically extended, and fortunately it is not a goal that longevity researchers are aiming for. However, it is a common concern when people are asked about the prospect of living longer.

As a reader of this book, you may be surprised that most people don't want to live forever. I certainly was. As someone who never has enough time to do everything I want, I've always considered death a major inconvenience to my continued enjoyment of life and I assumed everyone else saw it that way too. However, plenty of studies have found that most people don't want to live much beyond what is currently the norm, though I suspect this is more to do with them struggling to see past what may soon be possible, rather than a well-informed decision.

In 2013 a Pew Research Centre survey found that US adults considered an ideal life span to be 90 years, that's less than 10% more than how long people can expect to live, on average, right now. Over half of the respondents said they would not choose to undergo medical treatments to slow the ageing process, with less than one in ten people wanting to live longer than 100 years.

A more recent survey by Lifetime Daily found more than four in ten people wanted to live longer than 100 years. So, has public opinion shifted dramatically in those three years? I don't think so. One important difference with the Lifetime Daily question was that it assumed ageing stopped at 25, so people would live longer with the physique and energy of their 25-year-old selves.

The same has been demonstrated in other studies, where the desire for longer life increases with the option of living with a youthful body and/or mind, rather than with the prospect of living longer like a modern day senior citizen. David Ewing Duncan has been conducting an informal survey for many years now, asking attendees (totalling around 30,000 in total) at his talks how long they want to live. He says the results have always been reasonably consistent with only 10% wanting to live longer than 120 years. He also followed up with some of the people, who chose 80 years as their ideal lifespan, to determine the thinking behind their decision. The most common reason by far for not wanting to live more than the current average, was the fear of physical and mental decline.

These concerns are not new. In Greek legend, Eos (the Goddess of the Dawn) fell in love with Tithonus and asked Zeus to grant him eternal life so that they could live together forever. However, she forgot to ask for eternal youth as well, so he withers away until he can no longer move or lift his limbs. A lesson that no modern day longevist wants to repeat.

Longevity researchers are hoping that living longer in a young (or younger) body and with a sharp mind is the most likely scenario, as the underlying causes of ageing are discovered and treated. Everyone is looking to prevent or minimise suffering in old age and that will be the first step to eliminating old age entirely. Further steps, such as rejuvenation biotechnology, will eventually reverse the mental and physical damage caused by ageing, giving everyone the option of longer lives in a condition that makes it something worth living for.

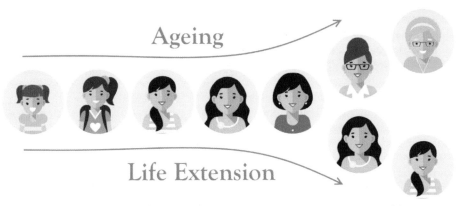

Rejuvenation biotechnology will reverse mental & physical damage caused by ageing

Life expectancy has jumped in a century

It's commonly said that life expectancy doubled in the 20th century. However, that is a global average so it takes into account the improved hygiene and diet that were already available to much of the US and Europe. Still, the UK saw an increase of over 50% in life expectancy between 1901 and 2001, and that has doubled since 1841. In the 19th century there was a much higher number of infant deaths which reduced the overall life expectancy, meaning that someone who made it to 20 in 1841, had a life expectancy of 60, only 20 years less than today.

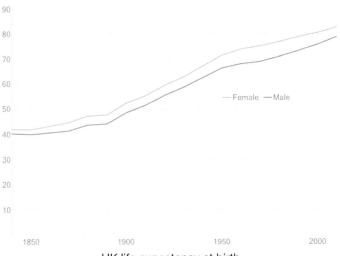

UK life expectancy at birth

Worryingly, this trend has started to slow down, reducing the long-term increase in life expectancy from 3 months a year to 1 month a year in the UK. The situation is even worse in the US with life expectancy falling for two years in a row, in 2015 and 2016, and making this the first drop since 1963. Research mainly blames this on an ongoing opioid epidemic, which has resulted in a 21% increase in overdose deaths. This does suggest this drop is likely to be a temporary blip, which has a political and economic solution rather than a medical one.

Surprisingly, if we were to cure cancer tomorrow that would only add about 2-3 years to life expectancy, because it's an average of everyone's lifespans and only relatively few people actually die from cancer. In the end, even if we cured all diseases using conventional treatments, life expectancy would struggle to rise much above the current maximum lifespan. This is because, slowly but surely, our cells just stop working meaning our organs and our body eventually die. A strategy to counteract that decay is discussed in *Curing ageing* and there are clues in nature as to where to look.

Immortal animals

Human life expectancy globally is 70 years which makes us one of the longest-living animals on the planet and almost doubles that of other primates. However, some tortoises are known to live longer and the bowhead whale has been known to live to over 200 years-of-age, making them the oldest mammals. Also in the sea, Greenland sharks only reach sexual maturity at 150 and can live for around 400 years. Though that is nothing compared to some simpler organisms such as escarpia laminate tube worms which may live for over a thousand years. What's more, these creatures are living in the harsh "survival of the fittest" natural environment – with no healthcare, government support or help when they get old – imagine how old they might grow if they were able to take action to live longer!

Typically, in the animal kingdom, the maximum lifespan varies and is strongly correlated with body mass, so larger species such as primates live longer than smaller species such as dogs. However, there are some outliers that live disproportionally long lives for their size.

The most famous example is the naked mole rat (or NMR to its fans) that lives nine times longer than other, similarly sized rodents. What makes the NMR interesting is that it is almost immune to cancer with very few cases ever reported. There are many possible reasons for this, including a more efficient DNA repair mechanism that minimises cell damage from mutations. NMRs also have higher levels of a cancer suppressing protein in their blood. Interestingly, the amount of this protein in human blood reduces with age, which may be one reason why we are more prone to tumours as we get older.

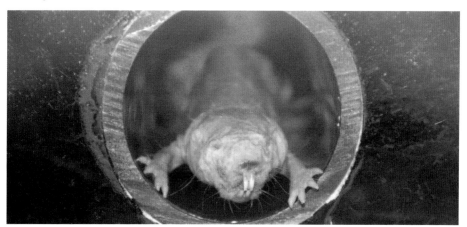

Naked mole rat

Other animals have the ability to regenerate themselves. Birds have the ability to repair damage to the inner ear and salamanders are able to regrow their limbs and tail. This process has been studied to see how a small clump of cells grow into new skin, muscle and cartilage. It appears that some cells, found just under the surface of the skin, are pluripotent, meaning they are able to develop into different types of cell. The hope is that lessons learnt from salamanders might lead on to stem cell treatments in humans to repair spinal cord injuries and grow replacement organs.

All of this ignores plants, which are living organisms with the same DNA structure that codes for some of the same proteins as humans. Many species of tree live thousands of years and one Great Basin bristlecone pine, which is still living in California, has been dated to 5,067 years.

All of these natural oddities are being studied to try to find their long-life genes and to discover any other mechanisms that help them defy ageing. In future, some of these biological components may become the basis for human anti-ageing therapies.

Should we?

We'll look at approaches to how ageing might be prevented in *Curing ageing*, but before we get onto that, it's worth discussing some of the common concerns raised when raising the prospect of living forever. Many of these worries may be gut reactions as the concept is likely to be totally new to most people, but once people have put more thought into it several familiar themes tend to emerge.

Unnatural

The most common argument is that life extension is simply unnatural. In my opinion this is possibly the most unformed argument, as it invites an open-ended discussion on what is natural. Across the animal kingdom, nature has evolved murder, infanticide and cannibalism as survival strategies, and however abhorrent we might find these behaviours it is difficult to classify them as unnatural. Similarly, if we are products of nature, how can anything we decide to do be considered unnatural? Steam power, electricity, and powered flight were all once viewed as unnatural, but most people wouldn't argue against their benefits today.

Putting that aside, let's look at the viewpoint that we would be tampering with nature. I agree that we would be changing how things are today, but the natural state of things is to change all the time. Species come and go (as I'm sure humans will) and have done so for millennia – over 90 % of mammal species were wiped out by an asteroid impact around 66 million years ago.

As we've seen above, life expectancy has recently doubled, so what is the natural lifespan of a human that we should defend and use medicine to try to achieve? It can be difficult to differentiate between where medicine is dealing with disease instead of "natural" ageing – where does the boundary lie? What should we do with medicines that cure a disease and, as a consequence, also push life expectancy up even more? Should these medicines be banned? We say people have "had a good run" if they get to their 90s because statistically that is the case at the moment – not because we have sat down and thought about how many years someone should live. Imagine if life expectancy doubled and people regularly lived to 200 – then when someone died at 90 we would think that was short-lived, in the same way we do if someone doesn't make it past middle-aged now.

Therefore, suggesting a moral maximum lifespan is picking an arbitrary number, and as we have seen with surveys of how long people want to live, it is often anchored to what is typical today. Surely, life extension can't be considered unnatural, at least until we are living longer than all the other animals.

Death gives life meaning

Another concern is that without death, life would be robbed of its meaning. This view goes back a long way. Although the ancient Greek gods were immortal they were considered by some to live somewhat shallow lives, which often only had meaning when they engaged with mortal humans. However, was this emptiness because of their immortality or maybe because, as gods, they already had everything?

Back on planet Earth the question is whether people with an indefinite lifespan would spend their time wisely? As there would always be time to do something in the future, it could always be put off until tomorrow or until the next century. How would our minds cope with planning a life that spans thousands of years? I imagine it wouldn't, but nor does it cope well with planning a few decades. Most people don't have a life plan set out in advance and it's very hard to predict what opportunities will or won't come along to change one's intentions. But, that doesn't mean people don't do things today just because they don't know what will happen tomorrow. I do things today because I enjoy them (or like most people to earn money to be able to do things I enjoy) which means I'm unlikely to postpone these experiences indefinitely.

One fear that I do agree with is that people would become risk-averse, as every decision would be risking forever rather than a few decades of deteriorating life. Would astronauts be less willing to take the 1 in 100 chance of dying per launch, would people take part in medical trials, would progress stall as fewer risks were taken? Who would enter careers that had any risk at all involved – police, fire brigade or armed services to start? But even outside of work, would life just become duller and duller with no-one willing to risk their indefinite lifespan for the thrill of a parachute jump, a horse ride or a simple swim in the sea? In Rachel Heng's book, Suicide Club, society is on the verge of biological immortality, and people are not only careful about what they eat and drink but also restrict what they listen to, so as to control their cortisol levels and prevent stress-related damage to their bodies. I have already taken one small step in that direction. In my forties, and already looking after my health, I realised that one of the biggest risks of death was a car crash – so out went the two-seater sports car and in came the slow but steady SUV - and I'm already looking enviously at newer models with more advanced safety features.

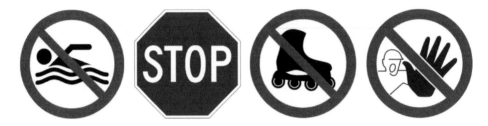

Would people stop taking risks?

One version of the "life needs death" viewpoint is that the transience of life is its most important aspect. This belief is summed up in Leon Kass' quote "Just as a pretty flower is beautiful because we know it will eventually wilt, the sunset is beautiful because it is short-lived." I observe the physical frailty of flowers and insects, the sweeping grandeur of landscapes and the mind-blowing wonder of galaxies but I've never considered the beauty of something to be a factor of its lifespan. Perhaps if the Earth was permanently swathed in a stunning sunset I'd get used to it and its beauty would wane, but that would happen over time rather than as a sudden decision that it no longer met my criteria for beauty after I had looked at it for a specific number of hours.

Boredom and the Loss of Self

This is probably the argument that I struggle most to relate to: that with so much time people would get bored and eventually have nothing left to do. Now for people who are enduring hard lives, who are working two or three jobs and still struggling to feed and protect themselves and their families, I can understand that the prospect of living longer is no big attraction, and I truly hope that as technology rapidly improves (see chapter on Exponential Improvements in Technology) the benefits will be spread more evenly, so that everyone is able to enjoy life. But I hear these arguments from the middle classes who, yes, are working, but have free time and the means to pay for leisure activities and travel. For me there are never enough hours in the day or weeks in the year to do everything I want to do. With a longer life I'd eventually be able to try all of the activities I've ever considered attempting and visit all of the places that makes the world so interesting. And I'd be able to speak the local language, when I got there, because I'd have at last had the time to learn it.

Would it eventually be possible to run out of things to do, even with an indefinite lifespan? I'm not sure this would even be the case with thousands of years of life, because as one lives, other people are also living and building and creating new art to appreciate, new activities to experience, and new places (perhaps even new planets) to visit. Bucket lists will just keep getting longer.

The structure of life will change too. Rather than the current norm of childhood, education, work and retirement, it is likely that education and work would turn into an ongoing cycle with people having multiple careers, and using the skills learned in one industry or speciality in another. We would be always learning and keeping the mind active with a pace of change tuned to the needs of the individual. Ethics will also need to change to accommodate the new reality. We'll adapt to longer lives with lifelong commitments becoming obsolete - for example, marriage. It would be improbable that two people would remain compatible over centuries of different personality changing experiences.

Combined with the "we'd get bored" argument is often the "we'd lose the sense of self" fear. This essentially says we'd be living for such a long time, and experiencing so many things, that we would no longer be able to remember what we'd done, who we'd met and more importantly who we are. The technoprogressives' answer to this quandary is that by then your brain will be so intimately connected to the internet that you'll have the extra memory and processing power on hand whenever you need it. However, I'll park that answer for now and address the problem based on a purely biological human. Would I, in 200 or 2,000 years' time, remember what I've done today and how I feel? No. But then again, I don't remember what I did twenty years ago or even two years ago, in detail, and have to put some thought into remembering what I was doing even two weeks ago. I have memories of fun incidents in my teens and twenty-somethings and I also realise how much I've learnt in the meantime, but I wouldn't choose to go back to being the same person I was then. However, I know that all of my choices, and therefore all of my experiences to date, have built me into the person I am today, and it is that person that I want to Preserve. This is true, even in the knowledge that that person will be slightly different in two years' time, in the same way as some of my views and opinions have slowly changed in the last two years.

You don't have to

The arguments against life extension discussed so far are areas where we have a personal choice. If someone strongly believes that humans should not live longer or past some arbitrary age, then there is nothing forcing that person to participate in whatever treatments, or to take whatever medicines are needed to keep them alive.

Anti-ageing treatments will not be forced upon people. Just as today there are conscientious objectors to some medical treatments and their wishes are respected, including Jehovah's Witnesses who don't accept blood transfusions and Hindus who avoid drugs and medical devices that contain parts of pigs or bovines. Likewise, when cancer patients decide the benefits of chemotherapy no longer counter its side effects and opt for palliative care instead. Doctors must respect a patient's decision even if they think it is wrong or irrational – in the future that should include life extension support, and doctors will not put pressure on patients to accept anti-ageing treatments.

Selfish

Life extensionists are often called selfish, arrogant, and narcissistic – but these just seem to be personal attacks on people with opposing views rather than arguments in their own right. Life extensionists may be working on and promoting something that is important to them, but that in itself does not make it wrong. So is life extensionism as a goal inherently selfish? Only, and according to its definition, if the people involved are thinking solely of their own advantage, and I don't think that is the case.

Most life extensionists believe that preventing disease and curing ageing is good for society and it isn't something they are trying to hoard for themselves. I see nothing selfish in trying to provide everyone with more health and more life. There are possible impacts that need to be acknowledged (see the "what if" chapter) just as there are with any new technology. Researchers in this field are probably more aware of the larger picture than most, as living forever doesn't only mean curing ageing, it also requires a stable society where people can live forever without fear of war, famine or the collapse of humanity. This makes them even more likely to ensure that everyone, if they want to, is able to benefit from their findings without keeping it for themselves, which seems the total opposite of selfishness.

It may be the tech billionaires who make the headlines when they invest in ageing research, but the scientists who are doing the work are generally working for basic salaries so are keen for cheap access for all when new treatments become available. Many of them give a lot of their time for free, to help raise awareness of the developments in ageing research and how new technologies will increase healthy human lifespans.

More important things

Another argument frequently thrown at longevists is that there are more important things to research. Agreed; there are always going to be limited resources available and agencies around the world try to share the available funds fairly. Depending on your point of view, different fields have a higher or lower priority but few would argue that even their personal preferred option should use all of the funds. Fusion power may provide cheap power to the world and solve a myriad of problems, but if we spent every science research dollar on that now, then there would be no money left for cancer or any other medical research. Of course, a cure for cancer would be fantastic, but if the hunt for its eradication soaked up all of the research budgets and scientists then there would be nothing left to tackle environmental issues, to develop new materials for batteries and transport infrastructure, or to keep enhancing the computer technology that has powered so many improvements in the last fifty years.

As an aside, the "couldn't you be doing something better" argument is one that is also used by people caught speeding – shouldn't the police be solving murders instead of prosecuting minor traffic offences? Well, of course murder is more serious, but life would be unbearable if every other crime was just ignored while officers only investigated offences where people have died. The same goes for scientific research.

So accepting that other studies need to continue, should anti-ageing research be receiving any funding at all from existing science budgets and investors? Or should the focus continue to be on specific diseases that cause suffering and death? Well, ageing causes suffering and death too, so why should it be relegated to behind other conditions?

As ageing is the underlying cause of most non-communicable diseases (i.e. those not caused by an infection) any discoveries are likely to have a knock-on effect for several chronic conditions, possibly saving money overall. For example, one approach to curing ageing is LysoSens (see Curing Ageing) and one of its first targets will be artery plaques which will reduce heart disease. Likewise, tissue engineering, which is a focus of medical rejuvenation, could save the lives of the thousands of people around the world, who die every year while waiting for an organ transplant.

But, what if?

What if longevists win the argument, secure enough funding for their research, and bring about radical life extension in the near future? It is fair to assume that the change will be so fundamental that it will have manifold effects on the world. If so, many people, including those who want to live longer healthier lives, may have legitimate concerns about the impact on themselves, society and the planet. Here I try to address a few of those worries and emphasise that most of them are not new problems, they're just current dilemmas applied to a new phenomenon.

Inequality

If you see life extension as a benefit, and possibly the greatest benefit of all time for humanity, then it's likely you would wish it to be available to all, in the same way as you'd like basic healthcare to be available to everyone across the globe. There is currently a big difference in healthcare provisioning between and within countries, so will the same happen with anti-ageing care?

Probably. The divisions and inequalities in the world today are unlikely to be affected by new anti-ageing treatments, but one can hope that in the same way as new technologies and medicines eventually trickle down to the less well off ("a rising tide lifts all boats"), then the same will happen with new therapies. Just as in the mass production of phones and pharmaceuticals, economy of scale should ensure medicines and treatments are available to all. Typically, most of the cost is in the research and development and, once patented, and ready for market, the biggest profits are made by selling to as many people as possible.

The big risk is that the advantages provided by radical life extension will widen the gap between rich and poor, particularly as the rich are likely to have access to the treatments sooner than everyone else, and before the costs fall enough to make them affordable for all. This advantage could allow the well-off to accumulate even more wealth, would be hoarded and unavailable to the benefit of society. As today, the distribution of wealth is a matter of public policy and so will be a problem to be raised with politicians who can make and change laws. Some of the current mechanisms that tackle inequality of wealth, for example inheritance tax, will no longer be appropriate when few are dying, so new laws and taxes will be needed to deal with the new reality.

Conversely, this risk may also be the biggest opportunity. In the UK the better off live eight years longer on average than those living in the poorest areas, which is about 10% of the average life expectancy in this country. But what if life expectancy was 160 instead of 80? Then that lifespan advantage would only be 5% and would be further reduced to 2% when we're living to 400. Eventually, when everyone is living forever, the advantage vanishes to nothing - nobody can live longer than forever!

Over population & limited resources

Another concern is that the population will grow uncontrollably and the planet will not be able to support it. Overshooting the available resources is already a concern and Armageddon has been foretold many times; ever since 1798, when Thomas Robert Malthus first predicted the human population would outstrip resources within 100 years. But there was no cataclysm in the 19th century, and even though the global population multiplied four fold in the twentieth century, grain production grew fivefold. This ensured there was enough food to go around, even if it was unequally distributed. More recently, in 1925, the head statistician for the U.S. Food Administration, Raymond Pearl, forecast that the U.S. could only support 200 million people, however that number was surpassed in 1938 (and is now 319 million). He was even further off the mark with his calculation about the carrying capacity of the whole planet, which he put at 2 billion people. That level was surpassed just a few years later. Even as recently as 1968, respected Stanford University professor, Paul Ehrlich, wrote "The battle to feed all of humanity is over. In the 1970s hundreds of millions of people will starve to death in spite of any crash programs embarked upon now."

These apocalyptic predictions were mainly based on the assumption that the global population would grow ever faster and that food production would not be able to keep up. In fact, what has happened since 1970 is that the rate of population growth has slowed steadily (although it is still increasing it is happening much slower) and the current United Nation's forecast is that it is most likely to plateau at just over eleven billion around the year 2100. As countries develop and families no longer need to rely on children for their labour or to provide care in their old age, fertility rates drop and in many countries they are already below the replacement level required to prevent the population falling.

Let's not forget that life extension is only able to provide *biological* immortality; people will still die in accidents, war and natural disasters, and based on current surveys a reasonable percentage of people will choose not to extend their lives. Governments will probably introduce regulations to restrict the number of children per person, along the lines of China's recent one-child policy. If the number of children allowed was two or fewer, even allowing for those children, and their children's children, there would still be a finite limit to the population the planet had to support.

The key resources that people need are food, fresh water and energy. It is the last of these that could provide new solutions for the first two, as new production methods may require extra energy, ideally from clean sources which are coming – see Exponential Improvements in Technology chapter for more details.

In the 20th century, food production outstripped population growth; but, eventually we will no longer be able to squeeze any more grain from a hectare of field. However, there are new ways to grow outside of existing fields – including upwards and downwards. Many researchers are looking into vertical farms which are super-efficient, clean and more environmentally friendly, as they don't require carbon intensive production methods, and can be located within cities, close to the consumer; thus, minimising the environmental impact of food miles. Growing upwards will allow more food to be grown per hectare. Likewise, the oceans have barely been scratched as a farming resource. Fishermen in the US, who have suffered from fish stock collapse and hurricanes, are investing in vertical underwater farming and reporting a yield of 25 tons of kelp and 250,000 shellfish per acre without the need of fertilisers or pesticides. Compare that to the US average for wheat of around 3 tons per acre, and the fact that oceans cover 70% of the planet. It's fair to say there is still plenty of capacity to increase food production. This should ensure that the (slowly) growing population can be fed for the foreseeable future.

So, is there a plan B, if we do start filling up this planet? In my article for the Institute for Ethics and Emerging Technologies I considered three options: we find more places to live on the planet, we each take up less room on the planet, or we find some more space off this planet. Building up and down would temporarily solve any problems of overpopulation; always assuming we can generate enough cheap and clean energy to power and cool the structures. Perhaps by then we won't all need as much space as we do today – if we plug in, Matrix-style, we'd only need a pod each. If you could have hundreds of times the knowledge and a thousand times the experiences by living in a virtual world I think there'd be some takers for that. Then the final option is colonising space – a topic many a movie has addressed; but is it realistic? Financially, at least, it is surprisingly so. NASA's Advanced Space Transportation Program aims to reduce launch costs to $200 per kilogram by 2025. This means that to dispatch enough people, to make room for the seventy-five million people born every year, would cost just over a trillion dollars. That's sounds like a lot of money but it's less than the amount the world spends on defence today. With a bit of effort, innovation and engineering there is no reason why an increasing population cannot be supported.

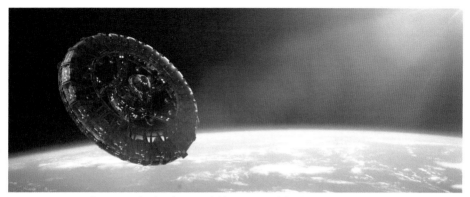

Space colonisation could be a surprisingly cheap option

Social impacts

What will be the impact on the structure of society when people live radically longer lives? Some practices rely on the steady churn of people getting older and dying. As the older generation retires, they create opportunities for the people below them to become the new leaders. However, if no-one dies then dead man's (shoes) jobs will never become available, amplifying the problem of incumbency. The current holder may be no better than those chomping at the bit to take over, yet it is hard to see how the, first come, first served, convention could be reversed. In business, innovation is key, so people and companies that stagnate will eventually fail, opening up opportunities for new directors and entrepreneurs. Of course, the flip side to this is that the world does not lose the minds holding decades of experience and knowledge, though this is of no recompense to those waiting below.

Then again, how much do we benefit from total life experience? Even with an indefinite lifetime, the brain only has so much capacity, so maybe we can only benefit from the skills and network connections used in the last, say, forty years or so and after then we will plateau. It may still be hard for people to break into an industry, but a 120-year old would be no better qualified than an 80-year old. So, as long as systems are setup as meritocracies, then the better people would excel – irrespective of their age. Though people might have more years in their lives, they will have no more hours in a day than anyone else. Therefore, although a person may wear many different hats over their lifetime, they can only wear so many hats at one time, limiting the amount of authority they can command.

What about public opinion? If there is a risk that organisations will stagnate, could society as a whole stagnate also? Nobel prize winning quantum physicist, Max Planck, once remarked, "A new scientific truth does not triumph by convincing its opponents and making them see the light, but rather because its opponents eventually die, and a new generation grows up that is familiar with it."

Like science, society also has big intergenerational differences of opinion on matters such as politics, race, sex and sexuality. In the UK there is a clear age factor in political allegiance. Ignoring (for convenience) the 10% that don't vote for the two main parties, roughly speaking only 20% of people under 25 vote for the right-leaning Conservative party, compared to 80% who vote for left-leaning Labour. However, by the time people are in their sixties this trend has reversed, which may be a warning that society will slowly align its political views as almost the entire population ages past 60.

Similarly, views on same-sex marriages are divided along age demographics. Pew Research in the US has tracked social views over time and has also broken them down by generation (e.g. boomers vs millennials). This is interesting because, as well as showing that support for gay marriage is much greater in younger people, the research also reveals that people born in a particular era have also changed their minds. So, unlike politics, where age is a factor, there is also an underlying tide of change that breaks through age barriers. This suggests that social opinion won't stall; but, just like today change takes time. Which, fortunately, we'll have plenty more of.

On more practical matters, society will have to think about whether the regulations and procedures it has in place today are still relevant when people are capable of living forever. For example, today, health and safety laws allow for a degree of risk balanced against cost; but, will the 100 workplace deaths a year in the UK still be acceptable when so many more years of employees' lives are at stake?

What about the criminal justice system? We will need to consider the impact of jail sentences on offenders – for those that regard incarceration primarily as a punishment, how effective is a ten-year sentence if life is never ending? Would this deter a career criminal who has unlimited time, outside of jail, to enjoy no matter how long he or she is inside? Perhaps sentences should include a prohibition on anti-ageing treatments in which case today's sentences may be too long because the loss of youthful years may be a greater punishment than the loss of freedom. Then again, perhaps after a prisoner is released it would only take an extra session at the nearest ageing therapy centre to get all those years back again! Perhaps new laws will be needed to restrict the amount of treatments ex-convicts can receive? This is going to be a complicated debate...

Individual morals may need to be adjusted also. It is generally accepted that in a disaster the children are saved first as they have more life remaining and therefore the most to lose, and this was reinforced in a recent Moral Machine study by MIT's Professor Iyad Rahwan. His team found that the four million participants overwhelmingly favoured the protection of younger lives. Assuming this logic is incorporated into self-driving cars in the near future, will it need to be adjusted when people live for thousands of years and the difference in lost years of life between hitting a 10-year-old or a 50-year-old is negligible?

Immortal dictators

What if dictators like Stalin and Mao had access to life extension treatments and were able to live indefinitely – would they also rule indefinitely? Stalin took over the leadership of the Soviet Union in the mid-1920s and ruled with an iron first until his death, in 1953, from a burst artery in his brain. During that time, he setup a life extension program at the All-Union Institute of Experimental Medicine and according to Bryan Caplan, professor of economics at George Mason University, would most likely still be ruling Russia today if it had succeeded in keeping him alive.

However, this argument is not applicable to all dictators. Many tyrants have been usurped because of internal power struggles, civil war, and military defeat, including Hitler, Mugabe, and Saddam Hussein. There is an argument that for some of those, who were seen off by their opponents, it only happened because they had already started to show the weaknesses of age. However, this needs to be counterbalanced with the question of would these dictators be able to put themselves into long-term positions of power, as easily, once death was no longer an option for their departure? Perhaps people would be less willing to accept titles such as "His Excellency President for Life" when life really meant forever.

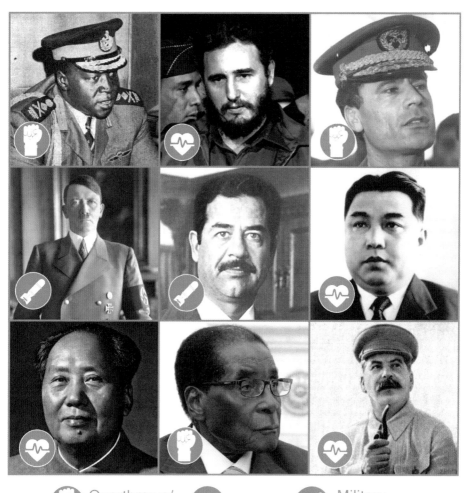

Overthrown/civil war — **Health** — **Military defeat**

Top left-to-right: Idi Amin, Fidel Castro, Muammar Gaddafi, Adolf Hitler, Saddam Hussein, Kim Il-sung, Chairman Mao, Robert Mugabe, Joseph Stalin

Dictators are unlikely to rule forever

What is ageing?

Most dictionaries define ageing along the lines of "the process of becoming old." In this context old isn't just the number of years that something has existed. No one talks about a diamond ageing or getting old – that's because it's structure and strength don't change over time. However, houses, cars and furniture age, not just in years but in functionality and appearance. Basically, ageing implies decline and deterioration.

The World Health Organization's "World Report on Ageing and Health" describes ageing as:

"The changes that constitute and influence ageing are complex. At a biological level, ageing is associated with the gradual accumulation of a wide variety of molecular and cellular damage. Over time, this damage leads to a gradual decrease in physiological reserves, an increased risk of many diseases, and a general decline in the capacity of the individual. Ultimately, it will result in death."

This general decline in function is also termed 'senescence'. Note that this refers to the whole organism (e.g. a person) and should not be confused with cellular senescence which is a specific cell-level activity that is discussed later.

The WHO's definition mentions "an increased risk of many diseases" which is a good way of keeping the definition of ageing as general as possible. There are plenty of statistics that show people's chances of suffering from particular diseases and ailments at different ages, but it's not possible to say exactly who will be afflicted with which one. However, it is safe say that the older people get the more likely they are to succumb to one or more life-threatening conditions.

Interestingly, this risk increases in quite a predictable pattern - your chance of dying doubles every eight years. At 40 years old a UK individual has a one in a thousand chance of dying that year. At age 48, that chance has increased to two in a thousand, and at 56 it's four in a thousand. This exponential increase in ageing is why, however lucky someone is with their genes and health, eventually, without the coming anti-ageing treatments, it will be impossible to outrun death.

There are hints that the risk of dying levels off for supercentenarians (people aged 110 and over), which means we stop ageing based on the above definition. However, by then people only have a one in two chance of surviving each year, so the possibility of even living to 120 are a thousand to one.

Underfunding

One of the reasons there is not a more precise definition of ageing is the historic lack of basic research; which can be partially attributed to the struggle for legitimacy and funding. Ageing research has always existed on the fringe of biomedical research, and is seen by many as a fanciful search for a fountain of youth. Therefore, it has therefore struggled to gain wider backing from the scientific community. Until recently, this has restrained ageing research to primarily a data gathering exercise with the manipulation of ageing as a niche within a niche.

In 2016, the US National Institutes of Health (NIH) allocated over five billion dollars to the National Cancer Institute, over $3bn to the National Heart, Lung and Blood Institute, and about only half of that to the National Institute on Aging, which includes funding research into Alzheimer's disease. So actual ageing research receives around 1% of the US science budget, which is typical around the world. What is surprising about this is that the total health costs of ageing have been estimated to be about 50 billion pounds (US$65bn) a year in the UK alone, so any research that could be translated to a longer healthspan would quickly pay back its investment.

Even though ageing is a driving factor in chronic disease, pharmaceutical companies

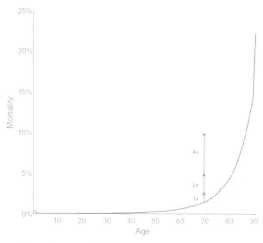

Your chance of dying doubles every 8 years

tend not to invest in the causes of ageing because the current healthcare business model is to pay for treatments for specific diseases. So even if they developed a pill that provided a few years' overall healthy life span, there is no mechanism for them to profit from it – much better to wait for someone to become ill and then sell healthcare providers a cure for that.

This is why some organisations have resorted to crowd funding, such as the Life Extension Advocacy Foundation. It has created its own funding platform (https://www.lifespan.io/) where it raises funds for projects, including screening compounds with the ability to block cancer pathways and AgeMeter – a device that estimates the biological age at which a person physically functions (i.e. functional biomarkers).

Others rely on commercial sales to fund their research. The Life Extension Foundation's corporate arm sells supplements and vitamins, and in its thirty-seven years of existence has provided $175m of funding into anti-ageing, rather than anti-disease, research much of which was awarded to projects for which it would be difficult to secure government grants.

One of the biggest organisations dedicated to age research, the Buck Institute for Research on Ageing, is half-funded by government research grants, with the other half of its budget supported by private donations and $6 million per year from the original Buck Trust Fund endowment. Its mission is to extend the healthspan with research into why ageing tissues lose their capacity to regenerate – the answer to which feeds into further research into how to target and prevent this loss. More on this later.

Biological Age

An inherent complication with ageing research is that people age at different rates. That's why we all live a different amount of time (our lifespan) which averages over the population as our life expectancy. Unlike in physics where a 1 kilogram ball will behave exactly the same as another 1 kg ball (under the same conditions), things are a bit more complicated with animals. Even identical twins with exactly the same DNA, upbringing and diet won't both experience the same diseases or die at the same time.

Each of us has both a chronological age, which is our age in years lived, and a biological age, which is determined by the health of one's body in comparison to the rest of the population.

Our biological age is affected by our genes, environment and lifestyle choices – only some of which we have control over. At the extreme end of bad luck genes is progeria – a genetic mutation that inflicts accelerated ageing on an individual. Children born with progeria have a life expectancy of only 14 years and often die of the same heart diseases suffered by most in middle-age. At the other end of the spectrum, we've all heard stories of 100 year-old people who have smoked twenty a day all their life and who still enjoy a large brandy – and they do exist – with good genes and a lot of luck. However, it is still a lot, lot more likely for someone to reach 100 by following some sensible advice – including the tips in this book!

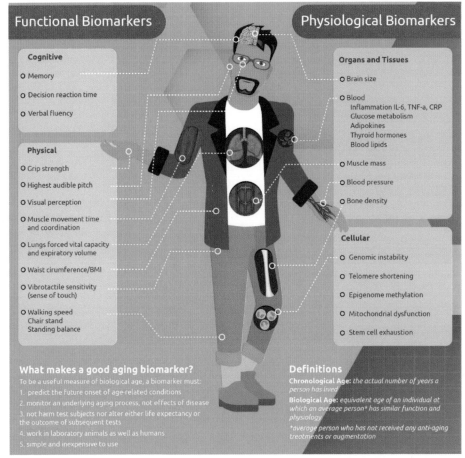

Functional Biomarkers

Cognitive
- O Memory
- O Decision reaction time
- O Verbal fluency

Physical
- O Grip strength
- O Highest audible pitch
- O Visual perception
- O Muscle movement time and coordination
- O Lungs forced vital capacity and expiratory volume
- O Waist cirumference/BMI
- O Vibrotactile sensitivity (sense of touch)
- O Walking speed Chair stand Standing balance

Physiological Biomarkers

Organs and Tissues
- O Brain size
- O Blood
  Inflammation IL-6, TNF-a, CRP
  Glucose metabolism
  Adipokines
  Thyroid hormones
  Blood lipids
- O Muscle mass
- O Blood pressure
- O Bone density

Cellular
- O Genomic instability
- O Telomere shortening
- O Epigenome methylation
- O Mitochondrial dysfunction
- O Stem cell exhaustion

What makes a good aging biomarker?
To be a useful measure of biological age, a biomarker must:
1. predict the future onset of age-related conditions
2. monitor an underlying aging process, not effects of disease
3. not harm test subjects nor alter either life expectancy or the outcome of subsequent tests
4. work in laboratory animals as well as humans
5. simple and inexpensive to use

Definitions
Chronological Age: *the actual number of years a person has lived*
Biological Age: *equivalent age of an individual at which an average person* has similar function and physiology*
*average person who has not received any anti-aging treatments or augmentation

Ageing biomarkers infographic – available online at https://go22.uk/biomarkers

Animal Models

Another difficulty with anti-ageing research is the length of time it takes to see the results of any intervention. Even treatment on people in their 60s will require at least two decades of follow up to see what the effects were on lifespan.

One way to get around this is to use an animal model (i.e. a non-human species) with a much shorter life-expectancy. Popular choices are Caenorhabditis elegans worms (c. elegans for short) and mice that have average lifespans of two weeks and two years respectively. As well reducing time, the use of animal models also significantly reduces the cost involved in experimenting on thousands of individuals, and also (to many) the ethical considerations. It's important to note that although the model organism may share some of the basic biology of humans, and even display the same symptoms when infected with a disease, any success seen in the laboratory is purely indicative until actually tried in a human. This is one of the reasons for the high cost of drug development – only one in ten drugs that start clinical trials are eventually approved, even after being proven in animals.

Hallmarks of Ageing

When looking at humans, there are physical changes that can be measured instead of waiting for people to die. Rather than analyse how long everybody in a trial survived, these changes indicate what effect the intervention is having and help predict the overall lifespan effect.

In 2013, a landmark research paper titled "The Hallmarks of Ageing" was published in the respected scientific journal, Cell, which identified nine underlying causes of ageing that accumulate throughout life. These hallmarks are summarised below, and then, in the following chapter, approaches to remedy them are discussed.

Genomic instability – this is damage to DNA caused by replication and other factors. DNA contains the instructions needed to build and operate all of the cells in the body. When cells divide (to grow or to replace dead ones) the DNA must be duplicated so that each cell has its own copy, however this can introduce errors into the code. More damage can also be caused by other natural agents, including sunlight and reactive oxygen species (free radicals).

Cells contain repair mechanisms that can either entirely reverse damage or minimise the loss of nucleotides (the individual letters of the DNA code). However, it is estimated that every cell in the body undergoes a million lesions per day, meaning that even with highly efficient repair machinery, not everything is repaired successfully and losses build up overtime.

Eventually the cell becomes so damaged that it triggers apoptosis – a form of beneficial cell suicide – but some become senescent (see below) or worse, cancerous.

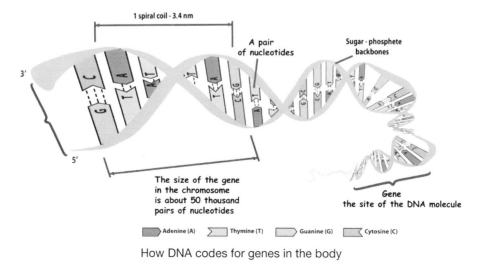

How DNA codes for genes in the body

Telomere attrition - telomeres are a special part of DNA that mark the ends of chromosomes (human DNA is packed into twenty-three pairs of chromosomes) and prevent them from fraying or sticking to other chromosomes. Unlike the random damage caused by genomic instability, telomeres tend to follow a more predictable deterioration.

When a cell divides the molecular machinery cannot work all the way to the end of the DNA strands and therefore the telomeres are left a little bit shorter each time. Eventually, after around fifty divisions (the Hayflick limit), the telomeres become too short and prevent the cell undergoing mitosis (i.e. dividing) again, and thus, these cells are unable to replace other damaged cells.

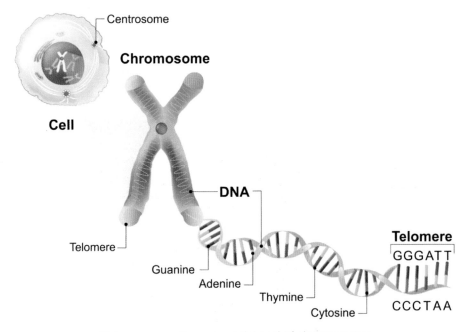

Telomeres are the caps at the end of chromosomes

Epigenetic alterations – these are detrimental changes to the way the DNA expresses itself, rather than to its code. Every cell in the body contains exactly the same DNA, however, it is able to build a variety of cells such as heart, skin, and liver. This is possible because DNA is not stored as one long strand but is wrapped around histones, and then coils itself into a fibre called chromatin. This physical structure means that some genes (small sequences of DNA with a particular function) are more available to be activated than others. So, even with identical DNA, cells can behave differently – this is known as epigenetics.

Methylation is a process that typically prevents genes that are not required by the cell from being used. However, this process starts to fail with age, compromising the cells metabolism and making the organ or tissue they are part of dysfunctional.

Loss of proteostasis – this is when the mechanism that regulates the synthesis and function of proteins begins to fail. Proteins are the building blocks of living cells and as well as providing their physical structure they also carry out most of the work. DNA can build about 20,000 different types of proteins to be used in the human body, with each gene coding for several amino acids, which then combine and fold up into a single protein.

It is the final shape of the protein that determines its function. So, if a protein folds

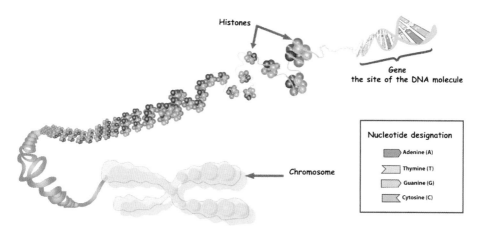

Histones

Gene
the site of the DNA molecule

Chromosome

Nucleotide designation

Adenine (A)
Thymine (T)
Guanine (G)
Cytosine (C)

The wrapping of DNA means genes behave differently in different cells

incorrectly the body tries to break it down and re-use its amino acids, or ejects the protein entirely. As well as being a contributing factor to ageing generally, unfolded, misfolded and aggregated proteins are known to cause specific diseases such as Alzheimer's and cataracts.

Deregulated nutrient-sensing – nutrient-sensing, as the name suggests, is the cell's ability to sense what nutrients are available for processing. To conserve energy, a cell only manufacturers molecules when it needs them and when fuel (e.g. glucose) is available to power their production.

Nutrient-sensing uses signalling between receptors on the cell membrane's surface and its nucleus, which affects the rate of cell growth and metabolism. Research suggests that dampening this signal extends longevity and therefore ways of artificially reducing it, such as calorie restriction, are a key area of study. However, if lowered too much the cell can stop functioning altogether – this is what happens to the levels of insulin-like growth factor 1 (IGF-1) during normal ageing.

Mitochondrial dysfunction - mitochondria are the parts within a cell that convert fuel into adenosine triphosphate (ATP) which is used to power the rest of the cell. Just like the engine in a car, even if the rest of the vehicle is in good condition, not much happens if it's not working.

As the mitochondria convert oxygen (O2) into ATP, sometimes an electron is accidentally released forming reactive oxygen species (ROS) that can damage the cell - and because of its proximity, this damage is likely to be to the mitochondria itself. Damaged mitochondria release even more electrons resulting in a positive feedback loop that reduces the efficiency of the energy production and also damages the surrounding cell, accelerating ageing.

Cellular senescence - this is the name for when cells stop replicating because of damage, or the cell reaches its Hayflick limit, or for a multitude of other reasons. Senescence itself can be a good thing, and in young damaged cells it makes sure they do not replicate and risk developing into cancer. As we age, these senescent cells start to accumulate as a consequence of both an increase in the rate of their generation and a decrease in the rate that they are removed.

Unfortunately, senescent cells don't just benignly take up space in tissue, they also excrete a whole range of pro-inflammatory signals. This senescence-associated secretory phenotype (SASP) encourages other cells to enter the same senescent state

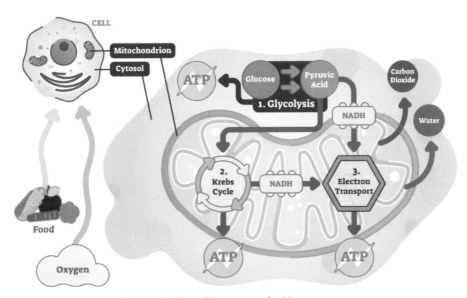

How mitochondria convert fuel into energy

and is also associated with many age-related diseases including type 2 diabetes and atherosclerosis.

Stem cell exhaustion – stem cells are cells that have not specialised into a specific type of cell (e.g. heart cell or skin cell) but are able to create new cells of different types. Until recently it was thought that stem cells were only located in bone marrow but in the last couple of decades they have been found in different tissues throughout the body. As well as dividing to replace damaged cells, some stem cells are needed to create cells that never replicate themselves (e.g. red blood cells) and therefore must be continuously produced.

Alas, even these wonder-cells eventually wear out, losing their ability to differentiate so reducing the total number of stem cells in the body. This contributes to many aspects of ageing, including immunosenescence which is the deterioration of the immune system caused by the diminished production of adaptive immune cells.

Altered intercellular communication – the final hallmark, identified in the research paper, involves the signalling between cells that is controlled by either the endocrine system (hormones) or the nervous system. One of the key causes of intercellular communication deterioration is inflammageing – the chronic inflammation that accompanies the ageing process.

When this signalling fails, the composition of the tissue surrounding the cells changes, affecting its mechanical and functional properties, and leading to poor tissue repair and degeneration.

In summary

If that doesn't all sound complex enough, it's made even more complicated by the fact that each hallmark may affect, or be affected by, the others. For example, mitochondria dysfunction can cause damage to the cell's DNA and if that damage is to IGF genes, then nutrient sensing will be impacted too. In reality, I've only touched the very surface of each of these hallmarks, every one of which is a specialist area that a scientist could spend their entire career working on; so, I apologise to them for summing it up into a few paragraphs.

Curing ageing

In the last few decades we have not discovered anything more fundamental than DNA, which is made up of four nucleotides that define how amino acids are built, and which in turn form the proteins that manufacture and control all the cells in the human body. We may not have discovered every signalling pathway yet, or understand what every protein does, or how they interact with each other, but we do seem to have all the pieces – and however complex the jigsaw may be, further study and increasing computing power will eventually allow us to solve it. So where do we start?

Plan of Attack

As we learn more about the causes of ageing, rather than specific diseases, the more targets we have to attack to try to stop, and eventually reverse it. The SENS Research Foundation has described seven fronts, each of which needs to be defeated to halt ageing in its tracks.

SENS stand for Strategies for Engineered Negligible Senescence which hints at its engineering approach to curing ageing. It sees ageing as a physical problem - yes, a very complicated one, but a problem that can be solved. The seven fronts it has identified are major classes of cellular and molecular damage, which are caused by the body's metabolic processes – i.e. staying alive. The term, Strategies for Engineered Negligible Senescence, was first used in Aubrey de Grey's 2008 book, Ending Aging, and the list is particularly encouraging as the most recent cause of damage was discovered in 1982; and since then no other category of damage has been uncovered, so it looks as if this list is as long as it gets.

The SENS Research Foundation does not claim to be able to prevent the damage being caused by the body's natural processes, nor that it is possible to cure all diseases that are caused by the unmanaged build up of this damage. Its strategy is to repair the damage caused by ageing while it is still at a trivial level (no one notices ageing damage accumulating in their twenties), thus preventing the accumulation that eventually causes causes disease and death.

This engineering approach to repairing damage also has the added advantage that we don't have to fully understand the processes of decay and ageing. If it turns out we were wrong about how particular damage occurs, or there are alternative mechanisms, it doesn't matter as long as we are able to clean up the damage. Of course, the better our understanding the more likely we are to come up with more and better ways of removing the damage, but not fully comprehending the problem doesn't stop us from getting started now.

Strategies for Engineered Negligible Senescence

Here are the seven identified types of ageing damage and the strategies to combat them, as well as some of the initial approaches to keeping them in check.

Making cancerous mutations harmless (OncoSENS)

As noted in the hallmarks of ageing, DNA mutations and epigenetic alterations can damage cells and lead to age-related disease and disability. The greatest damage happens when unwanted modifications cause a cell's replication mechanisms to run awry, resulting in uncontrolled growth – better known as cancer.

One characteristic that all cancers have in common is their ability to increase the length of a cell's telomeres – without which tumours could not grow. As a cell's telomeres shorten with every division, all cancers must have a mechanism for preventing them getting too short. The main method to do this is to produce telomerase – an enzyme that is needed in some specialist cells, such as stem cells, but which gets hijacked by cancerous cells to elongate their telomeres.

Initially telomerase-inhibiting drugs may prevent cancers from thriving, however due to their fast rate of mutation and division, some cells may find ways to avoid, block or breakdown those drugs. So, although these drugs could save many lives initially, SENS is already looking past them and towards a strategy it calls WILT, or Whole-body Interdiction of Lengthening of Telomeres. This would entirely remove the telomerase-creating genes from the body, thus preventing them from being exploited by cancer cells.

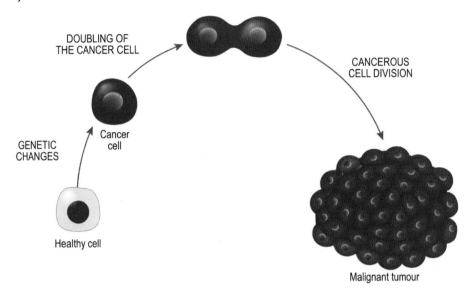

DOUBLING OF
THE CANCER CELL

CANCEROUS
CELL DIVISION

GENETIC
CHANGES

Cancer
cell

Healthy cell

Malignant tumour

Tumours are formed when cancer cells divide without limit

Preventing damage from mitochondrial mutations (MitoSENS)

DNA is held in a cell's nucleus, however mitochondria have some of their own, specialist DNA, called mtDNA. This mtDNA codes for just thirty-seven genes, compared to over 20,000 in the nucleus DNA.

As the mitochondria within a cell burn fuel to create energy, the free radicals given off by the process can damage mtDNA because of its close proximity to them. If the damage cannot be repaired, then the mitochondria are unable to produce the instructions required to tell the cell to create more proteins as it needs them.

The SENS proposition is not to try to prevent the damage, but to create backup copies of these genes. These backups would be stored in the main cellular DNA, away from the high-risk environment of the mitochondria. Over evolutionary timescales, around a thousand genes have already migrated from the mtDNA to the main nucleus, probably for the same reason, which means a mechanism already exists for the proteins to be imported into the mitochondria.

Removing dysfunctional cells (ApoptoSENS)

Dysfunctional in this sense means death-resistant cells. Usually when cells are no longer functional, or no longer needed, they go through a process called apoptosis where specialist proteins break down the cellular components into small pieces that can be vacuumed up and recycled.

The main types of dysfunctional cells are called senescent cells, as discussed in the hallmarks of ageing, and the good news is that although they build up over time, the actual number of senescent cells is low, which makes them a good target for slowing ageing. The two key ways to target these cells is either with a drug that is toxic only to senescent cells (by finding distinctive molecules that occur only on their surfaces) or to prime the immune system to seek out and destroy them even if they don't start apoptosis. There is already a lot of academic and commercial interest in these drugs, dubbed senolytics, with research in mice demonstrating that removing 30% of senescent cells slows down age-related decline and extends remaining lifespan even in older mice.

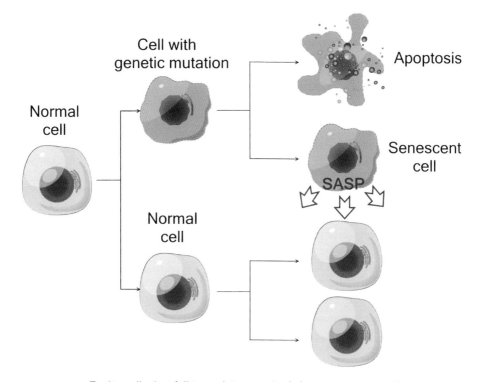

Faulty cells that fail to go into apoptosis become senescent

Replacing lost cells (RepleniSENS)

RepleniSENS is almost the opposite of the previous strategy, ApoptoSENS. Rather than getting rid of unwanted cells, its aim is to make sure the body doesn't run out of the cells that are needed. Around sixty billion cells die each day in the human body (that's about one in every thousand cells) because of molecular damage and physical trauma. They are replaced by new cells that are created when stem cells divide and differentiate into the required specialist cell type. However, over time this pool of stem cells becomes depleted and the remaining ones don't function as efficiently. Depending on their location, this can result in various conditions such as loss of strength (muscles), cognitive decline (brain) and reduced immunity (thymus).

The approach being taken to tackle this problem is to try to convert mature cells (i.e. ones that have already grown into specialised cells such as skin or blood cells) and to restore them to the state of a stem cell. These come in various levels of usefulness, from unipotent stem cells which can only create one type of specialised cell through to pluripotent stem cells (iPSCs) which can differentiate into nearly all types of cell. The next step is to produce as many cells as are needed, for example to repair the damage caused by a heart attack. A pharmaceutical company in Japan (Sumitomo Dainippon Pharma) opened a factory in March 2018, to do just that and to sell those cells for commercial applications.

One of the first applications of this technology will be growing new organs where they have failed, reducing the thousands of patients each year who currently die while waiting for a suitable organ donor. Because the cells have been grown from the patient themselves there is also no risk of the organ being rejected.

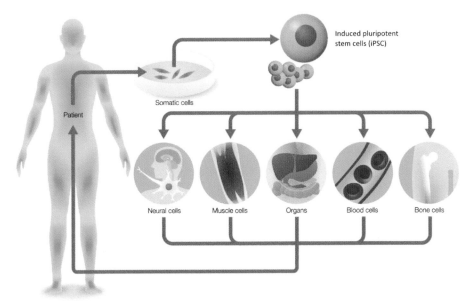

Stem cells from a patient's body can be replicated and used in regenerative medicine

Clearing waste accumulations out of cells (LysoSENS)

Intracellular junk is the aggregation of proteins and other biomolecules within the cell that are damaged or dysfunctional by the day-to-day biochemical accidents that occur during normal metabolism. This being a common occurrence, cells already have a built-in mechanism to handle this junk – the lysosome. Lysosomes work a bit like an acid bath – whatever goes in is dissolved by its multiple degradative enzymes - and the resulting products (sugars, amino acids and nucleotides) are released back into the cell ready to be incorporated into new macromolecules and organelles.

Some aggregates are so large that they cannot be broken down, often rupturing the much needed lysosome. As these accumulate they impair the function of the cell, eventually destroying it.

Macrophages are a particular type of lysosome, some of which consume the toxic by-products of cholesterol in blood. When these macrophages fail to break down the debris, they become immobilised and form plaques in the arteries, which leads to heart disease. Lysosome failure is also a key factor in several types of neurodegenerative diseases (e.g. Parkinson's and Alzheimer's) and in macular degeneration in the eyes.

The hunt is on for enzymes that will allow lysosomes to breakdown these larger or more stubborn molecules. Fortunately, we know they exist because without them human corpses would not be broken down; so the first place to look is in soil bacteria and fungi. Once these enzymes have been identified they will need to be tweaked to work inside the human cell. This may sound complicated (and it is!) but enzymes are already being successfully transplanted into patients with genetic disorders (e.g. Gaucher's disease) through enzyme replacement treatment (ERT).

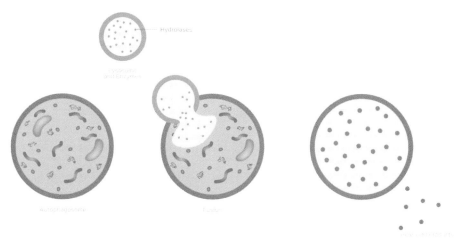

Lysosomes already recycle cellular waste

Removing junk from between cells (AmyloSENS)

Rather than dealing with the junk inside cells, AmyloSENS focuses on extracellular aggregates, i.e. the junk outside of cells. Even though it is not within a cell, extracellular junk can still impair the function of the tissue that the cells make up and can also disrupt organ structure.

Amyloids are accumulations of malformed proteins that clump together to form long fibre structures called fibrils. A well-known example of these abnormal clumps are the beta-amyloid plaques that build up in the brains of Alzheimer's patients. Amyloids are also a factor in type 2 diabetes and senile cardiac amyloidosis.

The solution to amyloids is to use specialised antibodies that home in and remove them from the tissue. Several companies are working on this including NeuroPhage Pharmaceuticals that uses its General Amyloid Interaction Motif (GAIM) platform to target multiple malformed proteins, and Covalent BioScience that has four catalytic antibody ("catabody") products in development. It may be that some malformed proteins cannot be dismantled with drugs, so researchers at Dundee University are also developing an Affinity-directed PROtein Missile (AdPROM) system that uses smaller nanobodies to target and bind to proteins enabling them to be destroyed.

Breaking extracellular crosslinks (GlycoSENS)

The final class of damage identified by the SENS Research Foundation are the unwanted crosslinks that build up between fibres in the extracellular matrix (ECM) – this is the network of collagen and other proteins that provides structure to tissues, and makes up around 25% of the body.

Occasionally, when blood sugar molecules pass through the matrix, they react with its protein fibres (such as collagen) creating chemical bonds – these are the so-called crosslinks. These connections restrict the flexibility of the scaffolding and can also alter the way nearby cells behave, because they use the stiffness of the ECM to guide their behaviour.

One consequence of this is that the matrix is unable to buffer the surge in blood passing through the blood vessels with every pulse of the pumping heart. The pressure is therefore trapped inside the arteries, raising systolic blood pressure, and allowing it to be carried directly to critical organs, putting them at risk of damage.

Because these crosslinks have very unusual chemical structures they are a good target for drugs to identify and attack, ideally reacting only with the unwanted couplings and severing them, without damaging any of the surrounding structure. Researchers have already discovered a drug that substantially lowers blood pressure in ageing animals - unfortunately, it has minimal impact on humans, but the hunt is on for human-specific crosslink breakers.

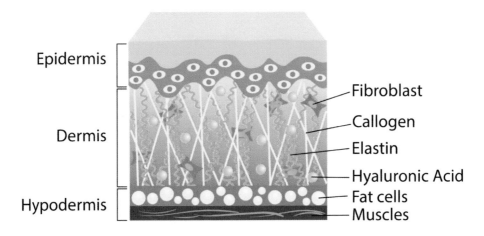

Breaking crosslinks in the skin's extracellular matrix will restore its suppleness

Reversing ageing (rejuvenation)

Just as with the hallmarks of ageing, this list of SENS' targets is only a summary of what teams of researchers are looking into, the detail of which is unbearably complicated and so better left to the scientists. What is important to us, the general public, is that it is happening, that there is a plan, and that progress is being made.

One worry that some people may have is what if I'm already old? Or, what if I'm middle-aged now, and will already be suffering from the effects of ageing by the time it can be stopped? Well, the good news is that the strategies outlined above will not only stop ageing but reverse it too. Often rejuvenation will use the same technique(s), only applied to a greater extent.

For example, with extracellular crosslinks, initial treatments will reach the easiest to find connections which are likely to be newly created ones, so regular treatments would stop this element of ageing. But to rejuvenate the tissues we'll need to develop treatments to track down the deeply buried crosslinks, and remove all of those as well.

No doubt as we start knocking off the already identified causes of ageing, new more subtle ones will emerge – though by definition these will work more slowly and allow us more time to research and tackle them. We just need to keep one step ahead, slowing down (and repairing) ageing damage fast enough to live a little bit longer, so that another therapy can be developed to tackle the next ageing mechanism. This is known as the longevity escape velocity.

Life extension glossary

There are many terms used in the discussion of living longer. Many of these are established scientific terms and therefore have clear definitions; however, some are newer concepts, which are still being developed, so their use may be less consistent, and their meaning may change over time.

Ageing - gradual biological deterioration that increases an organism's mortality rate (i.e. chance of dying) over time.

Biological Age – the equivalent chronological age of an individual, based on their current risk of death as determined by a variety of biomarkers.

Biological Immortality – human state once ageing has been cured and risk of death from disease or infection is negligible, but still subject to death from accident, natural disaster and human conflict (aka **physical immortality**).

Chronological Age – number of years that have passed since an individual was born.

Digital Immortality – replicating consciousness in a computer (aka **mind uploading**). No longer subject to biological weakness, however immortality is still not guaranteed given the risk of a technical failure.

Escape Velocity - when scientific breakthroughs are extending life expectancy by more than twelve months every year, i.e. fast enough that we can escape the pull of biological demise. Note that between 1911-2011 the life expectancy at birth in the UK increased by over three months every year.

Healthspan – the duration of an individual's life spent in a healthy state. Currently the UK average is around 64 years.

Immortality – a fictional concept where individuals, creatures or races cannot be killed (or only in a very specific way), for example Dorian Gray, vampires and Highlander.

Indefinite Life Extension – see biological immortality

Life Expectancy – the average age, within a given population, that people will live to. Currently this is 70.5 (68.3 males, 72.7 females) globally, 81.2 (79.4, 83.0) in the UK and 79.3 (76.9, 81.6) in the US. Note: this can also be specified for a particular age (e.g. 65) rather than at birth.

Life Extension – research and practice into extending human lifespan by slowing, and eventually halting, biological ageing. Sometimes prefixed with "radical" to emphasise its use of technological solutions (e.g. bionic organs) over purely biological methods.

Lifespan – actual amount of time an individual lived before death.

Living Agelessly (aka **negligible senescence**) – when an individual no longer ages. Note, however, that if an 80-year-old stopped ageing today, their current level of physical damage would give them a one in twenty chance of dying each year, therefore only a 1 in 500 chance of surviving to be 200 years old.

Longevity – a subset of a population who are predisposed to living longer than average.

Maximum Lifespan – the maximum amount of time an individual member of a population has ever lived. The oldest verified human was Jeanne Calment, a French woman who died in 1997, and who lived to 122 years and 164 days.

Radical Life Extension – see Life Extension

Rejuvenation – reversal of the mental and physical damage caused by ageing; enabling those with a high chronological age to become youthful again.

Senescence – see Ageing.

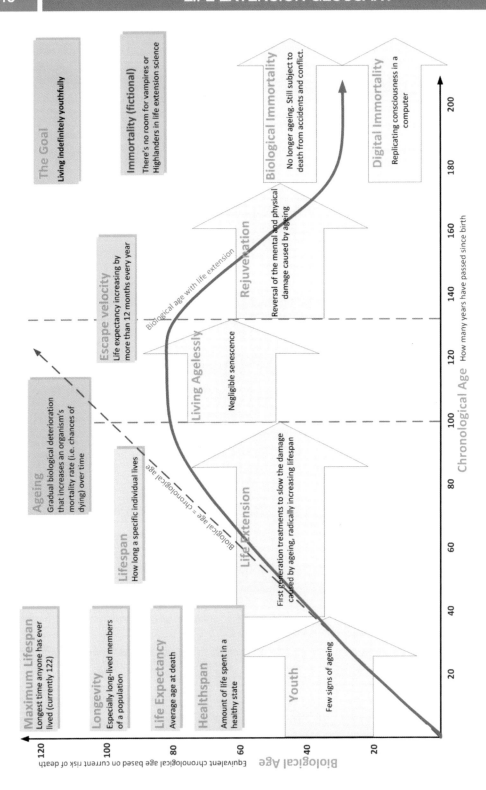

The Goal
Living indefinitely youthfully

Immortality (fictional)
There's no room for vampires or Highlanders in life extension science

Biological Immortality
No longer ageing. Still subject to death from accidents and conflict.

Digital Immortality
Replicating consciousness in a computer

Escape velocity
Life expectancy increasing by more than 12 months every year

Rejuvenation
Reversal of the mental and physical damage caused by ageing

Biological age with life extension

Living Agelessly
Negligible senescence

Ageing
Gradual biological deterioration that increases an organism's mortality rate (i.e. chances of dying) over time

Lifespan
How long a specific individual lives

Life Extension
First generation treatments to slow the damage caused by ageing, radically increasing lifespan

Biological age = chronological age

Maximum Lifespan
Longest time anyone has ever lived (currently 122)

Longevity
Especially long-lived members of a population

Life Expectancy
Average age at death

Healthspan
Amount of life spent in a healthy state

Youth
Few signs of ageing

Chronological Age   How many years have passed since birth

Biological Age   Equivalent chronological age based on current risk of death

120   100   80   60   40   20

20   40   60   80   100   120   140   160   180   200

Outrunning death

Let me be absolutely clear – the technologies required to provide biological immortality (that is, to prevent ageing) are not here today, and the discoveries needed to fix all aspects of ageing will not arrive in the next few decades either. Surely that means that anyone with only a few of decades of life expectancy remaining has no chance of living forever? No. What it means is that as each anti-ageing treatment arrives it will slow down the biological ageing process, buying a few more years, during which time another treatment will have been developed which slows it down a bit more, and the next one a bit more, and on and on.

Imagine the Grim Reaper, scythe in hand, steadily coming towards you. In your youth, you can easily outrun it, opening up a huge gap between you and termination. Inevitably, as you get older you start to slow down, but the Grim Reaper doesn't – it starts reducing the gap between you. Fortunately, you reach the first water station on this marathon of life and it has a special drink for you – maybe a small glug of senolytics that clears out some of your senescent cells, reinvigorating your muscles so that you can stretch that gap a little bit before you start slowing down again. Death starts to gain ground again, but once more you reach a water station, this time maybe the fluid has a recently developed enzyme in it that eats away and removes artery plaques, helping you avoid a heart attack during the race and it also boosts your energy so you get a little bit further ahead again. So even though Death will always be steadily coming for you, you just have to make sure you reach the next rejuvenation station before it reaches you. As the exponential growth in technology (discussed in the next chapter) means the development of new therapies will come at a faster and faster rate, meaning more frequent stations that allow you to keep comfortably ahead of the hooded slayer.

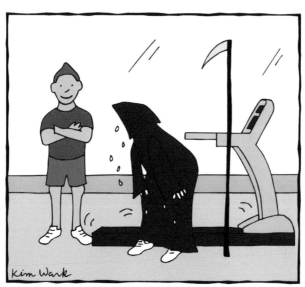

"Stop! You're killing me!"

Getting a head start

How do you maximise your chances of still being alive when the first generation of treatments arrive? How do you make sure that gap between you and Death is as big as possible so when you start to slow down you've got more time to reach the next revitalisation point?

Currently in the UK life expectancy is 81 years and 2 months but there is a wide variation in lifespan. Although the average is 81, around one in five people die before they're 70, and one in five people survive to be 90 or more. So how can you make sure you are in the 20% of people with a twenty year head start in the race against death?

Happily, you've made a good start by buying this book – the Live Forever Manual is your guide for getting ahead and staying ahead. Of course, buying the book is the easy part – following the tips takes a bit more effort.

It's not all in your genes

Some people may think it's not worth making the effort because they have bad genes, or truly believe that genetic make-up is more important than personal habits. However, research studies regularly show that lifestyle has a greater impact, and that genes have no more than a 25% impact on how long people live.

There are estimated to be between 300–700 genes that influence longevity, which would all have to line up in your favour to provide a major extension to your lifespan. It is more likely that some genes give an advantage and others a disadvantage, for example one gene may make you more susceptible to heart attacks but another may reduce your risk of diabetes. Hence one of the tips is to get a DNA test to see which diseases you are personally predisposed to, so that you can focus your preventative actions in that area. Likewise, if a particular condition runs in your family then you could put some extra effort into whatever lifestyle choices minimise your chances of suffering from that.

It's never too late to change your lifestyle. It has been shown that people who already have coronary artery disease, and are aged over 65, are able to lower the danger of an actual heart attack by up to 45%. You only have one chance to live forever so take action now!

How to become a classic

Another way to look at life extension parallels the way car enthusiasts look at classic models. Not many vehicles from the 1930s have survived eighty years of wear and tear but a few have been maintained so scrupulously that they look the same today as they did in their prime.

The renovators of these cars don't have to understand all of the chemical and physical processes behind each of the components of decay that send most motors to the scrap heap. They only have to know how to repair that decay and have the commitment to regularly check for and repair it again, and again, and again.

Similarly, the SENS strategy for damage limitation doesn't require medics to be able to stop ageing entirely. The human body already has several built-in repair mechanisms, such as enzymes that fix DNA level damage, lysosomes that clear up at the cellular level, and wound healing at the tissue level. Much of the early life extension research is looking at how these mechanisms can be improved or prolonged when they themselves start to fail.

Going back to some of the concerns people have about ageing treatments, their cost, and whether they will be available to everyone; I see another analogy with car restoration. Today, if you wanted your annual car service to include removing every minor rust spot and dent then it would end up costing thousands of pounds instead of a few hundred. That's because at the moment there is no demand for it, and the garage would need to bring in a specialist to do the job, so only a few people could afford it. But imagine if suddenly everybody decided to keep their vehicle in tip-top condition – immediately more providers would appear, competing with each other and driving down cost. Other companies would spring up to offer new tools and techniques for them to reduce prices even more, until reviving all of the body work might cost the same as replacing the brake pads.

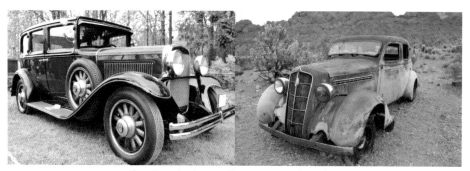

Continual rejuvenation vs natural ageing

Ship of Theseus

For those philosophically minded readers, the classic car analogy may itself appear as an analogy of the Ship of Theseus – a thought experiment concerning a ship, which has had all of its components replaced over time (as wood rotted and broke) – does it remain fundamentally the same object? The Ship of Theseus is already part of the discussion of human identity and existence, even before we start living forever, because most cells in the body are regularly replaced – begging the question that if "you" now are made up of entirely different atoms than "you" seven years ago (the average time it takes for cells to be replaced in the human body) what exactly is "you"?

Exponential improvements in technology

As explained in the Outrunning Death chapter, radical life extension is dependent on new medical technologies being developed faster than ageing creeps up on us, which means finding more and more treatments to keep slowing down the ageing process and repairing the damage already caused. Given the number of deaths every year from diseases such as cardiovascular disease and diabetes, why should we be optimistic that this rapid improvement is imminent?

Well, the concept of evidence-based medicine (i.e. based on comprehensive research) was only introduced, as an alternative to the then accepted practice of clinical judgement – i.e. based on the doctor's experience and intuition, in an academic paper in 1992. Unfortunately, intuition can often be wrong and be swayed by personal experience that does not reflect the best practice. For example, if a doctor treated a patient with a drug and that patient recovered, it would seem reasonable to that doctor to treat other patients who presented with the same symptoms with the same drug. This, even though that drug may not have been the cause of the recovery in the first patient and it may be responsible for long term harm. This sort of statistical proof can only be obtained through large-scale trials and monitoring beyond the resources of a single doctor. Until recently, healthcare has been as much an art as a science.

A good example of this is tonsillectomy – what used to be a very common practice of removing children's tonsils in cases of recurrent throat infections and tonsillitis. To the surgeon it would have made sense, because after the procedure the number of throat infections did reduce. However, the number of tonsil-related diseases in children naturally reduces with age, with or without surgery, partly because the tonsils themselves shrink after around age 6. Today, the number of tonsillectomies has dropped significantly, as not only are most unnecessary, but there is new evidence showing that the tonsils are an important first line of defence in the immune system.

As an aside, this is the same fallacy as people fall for at home with many natural remedies – self-prescribers take a bewildering number of different pills and potions for the common cold, and credit them when the cold goes away (spurred on by the companies that are making a healthy profit from these "cures"). However, people forget, or don't realise, that the common cold typically subsides a few days after the worst symptoms with no treatment whatsoever.

Linear v Exponential Growth

Research into health and the development of new drugs has been a slow and steady business for the last few centuries, and has followed a linear growth rate during that time. However, this work has recently started merging with (or at least being supported by) information technology, which allows it to benefit from the exponential growth in that industry. So, what is the difference between linear and exponential growth?

In summary, linear growth means increasing at a fixed rate, whereas exponential growth is when the amount of the increase also grows over time. This is a difficult concept to get your head around, and warnings about our failure to comprehend the extreme rate of growth have been around for centuries. In the legend of the Ambalappuzha Paal Payasam, the Indian god, Krishna, appeared as a sage to a king and challenged him to a game of chess. His prize, should he win, would be a few grains of rice – just one on the first square of the board, two on the second, four on the third - and the number of grains of rice keep doubling on each of the sixty-four squares on the board. It would be easy for someone to imagine that it could amount to a few sacks of rice, maybe, at most, a few carts, so the king readily agreed. When he lost, the rice was slowly presented – the last square on the first row of the board had only 256 grains, and at the end of the second row still only about 1 kg of rice was needed. But as the graph below shows, exponential growth starts off deceivingly slowly. The last square of the third row required 6 sacks of rice and by the end of the fourth row it was nearly 2,000 sacks of rice. By then, and with the board only half completed it was obvious the reward could not be met. To have delivered on his promise the king would have required several trillion sacks of rice.

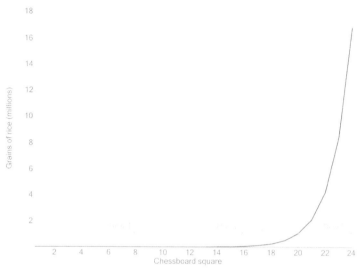

Doubling the grains of rice on a chessboard quickly gets out of hand

Moore's Law

The power of computers has been doubling, reasonably reliably, every two years for the last four decades. Gordon Moore was the co-founder of Intel and, having noticed a regular increase over a decade, predicted in 1975, that the number of components per integrated circuit would double every two years, thereby increasing the power and reducing the cost of computing. This observation has become known as Moore's law, and its consequences continue today, in supercomputers as well as consumer electronics, such as phones which keep on improving year upon year and getting cheaper and cheaper.

I remember the first USB memory sticks coming out with 8 MB of memory – and then doubling the year after to 16 MB. But we wouldn't be impressed if today's 256 GB memory sticks (a GB is 1000 MBs) were upgraded next year to 256.008 GB which would be the equivalent – no, we'll expect 512 GB memory sticks to be available – that would take 32,000 years to reach if capacity increased linearly.

The death of Moore's law has been predicted for almost as long as it has been observed. Technologists have said that it would not be possible to manufacture components smaller than 45 nanometres (achieved in 2008) or that physical laws would prevent them being reduced to under 10 nm (achieved in 2017). For every news story I read saying that Moore's law is coming to an end, I read another one with a new technology (such as optical and DNA computing) that could soon replace, and improve upon, existing transistor technology. The market will keep pushing for advances, because someone is always willing to pay a little bit more for a computer that is bigger, better and faster than their competitors.

So computer processors and memory are getting smaller, but what impact does that have on practical applications? Ray Kurzweil says it will be like experiencing 20,000 years of progress (at today's rate) within the 21st century. Though I'm not sure that really helps as 20,000 years ago homo sapiens were still in the Stone Age and imagine asking one of them what the world would be like now – probably just bigger and better things made of stone. Another way to look at it, and another Kurzweil prediction, is that by 2045, a supercomputer will have been built that is one billion times as powerful as, not just a human brain, but all the human brains on the planet.

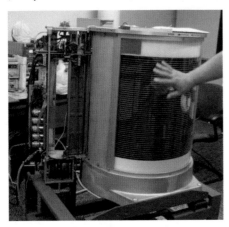

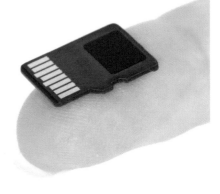

1956: IBM 350

2018: Micro SD

3.75MB ~US$75,000 (=$20m/GB)

256GB ~US$11 (=$0.04/GB)

The cost of memory has halved in price every 2 years for 60 years

A good example of how exponential growth has had a real-world impact is DNA sequencing. Not only has its cost reduced dramatically, but the applications have expanded beyond what was initially imagined. Early use of DNA analysis focussed on single gene disorders and required large budgets to research relatively common conditions. Now people can pay a few hundred pounds to get their own DNA tested for susceptibility to physical and mental diseases; individual cancers can be tested to determine their molecular weaknesses and patients can receive personalised medicine where the drugs they are prescribed are a better match for their DNA make-up and therefore more likely to be effective. Outside of healthcare, the costs are now low enough for DNA sequencing to be used in food safety, evolutionary biology and wildlife conservation.

In 1990, the Human Genome Project began, with the goal of sequencing the entire human genome, although it wasn't without its critics. Some called it "intellectually questionable" and claimed it would generate "enormous reams of uninterpretable and often useless data." Half-way into the fifteen-year project, some were still concerned as less than 1% of the genome had been sequenced by that time, but those attackers were falling for the linear fallacy and forgetting that 100% is only seven doublings from 1%. In fact, the project completed two years early.

As well as the speed of reading DNA being improved, the cost has also plummeted. One day after the end of the Human Genome Project, in 2001, Craig Venter's Celera Corporation sequenced the human genome for around $300 million. By 2006 that cost had dropped to $14m and by 2016, companies were offering to sequence entire genomes for $1,000 – that means it halved in price every six months.

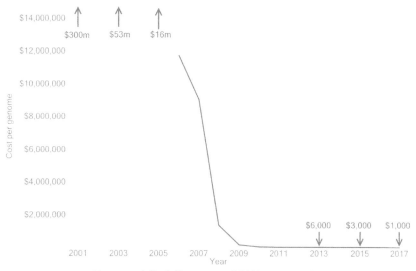

Exponentially falling cost of DNA sequencing

The Singularity

The exponential growth observed over the last century, loyally following Moore's law, shows how rapidly technology has advanced, and continues to do so, with any exponential graph eventually appearing as a vertical line as the y-axis value increases so quickly. This virtual cliff tends to act as a barrier to foretelling the long-term impacts of technological progress.

In 1910, around 38% of people were employed in the primary sector (e.g. agriculture, fishing, mining) and 30% were employed in the secondary sector (mainly manufacturing and construction) - that's a total of 68% of the workforce. Imagine telling them that in 100 years' time less than 15% of people would be working in those sectors – there would be panic and predictions of mass unemployment as what would the 53%, who lost their jobs, do? An economist may have predicted that other ways of working would evolve, but it would have been impossible to describe them at the time – how could they have imagined roles such as web designers, renewable energy consultants and coffee baristas that provide gainful employment today?

Likewise, the approaching robotics revolution is raising voices warning of job losses in the transport and retail sectors. There probably will be; it just ignores the new (and as yet unknown) types of jobs that lie around the corner. Perhaps the hospital cleaner, who has been replaced by a robot, will be retrained to be a team leader – not controlling the single robot that usurped him/her, but a small army of cleaning robots that are cleaning more areas, more frequently, than was economically possible previously.

What about beyond the just-about foreseeable future? When, in forty years' time, computers are a million times more powerful than today? Back in the 1950s, John von Neumann was one of the world's foremost mathematicians and pioneered the architecture that is still used in digital computers today. He observed the "ever accelerating progress of technology and changes in the mode of human life, which gives the appearance of approaching some essential singularity in the history of the race beyond which human affairs, as we know them, could not continue."

What he meant by that, and what has become known as the singularity, was that at some point in the future, technology will be improving so rapidly that humans will not have the ability to understand or control it. Up until now the acceleration of technological progress has been limited by the basic intelligence of the human brain, but we're already using technology to overcome that limit. No single person understands the full complexity of the hardware and software used in supercomputers, however they can be built and operated because of the technology leveraged by the whole design team. Soon the supercomputers themselves will be leveraging other technology to create even more powerful computers.

Of course, this is still expensive today, but don't forget the impact of exponential growth in technology. The EU's Human Brain Project was approved in 2014, with a budget of $1 billion and a ten-year project plan – a little less on both counts than the Human Genome Project. Its goal is to create a model of a working human brain and to simulate it on a supercomputer, starting down at the neurons and the electrical signals passing between them, up through the brain's sub-structures all the way to the two hemispheres. With the cost of computing power halving every two years, it will be twenty years after that (around 2044) that a $1,000 laptop could match human level intelligence.

This ties in well with the current thinking amongst AI researchers and futurists that the singularity is most likely to occur before 2050. In his 2005 book The Singularity Is Near: When Humans Transcend Biology, Ray Kurzweil examines past technological progress, and compares this against the computing power needed to exceed all biological human intelligence combined. He comes up with a date of 2045. Kurzweil has always based his predictions on the well-established curve of reducing computing costs, and has had a good level of success, such as in 1990 when he predicted that computers would beat the world's best players by the end of the decade, which they did. Give or take a couple of years, he has also predicted the arrival of touch screens, exoskeletons, and driverless cars.

As to what happens post singularity, this is one of the few areas where I tend to disagree with Kurzweil's vision and side with other thinkers such as Stephen Hawking and Elon Musk, who have warned that artificial intelligence could end mankind. Whilst acknowledging that it's imperative to get it right first time, Ray suggests in his book that the free-market system "will provide the most constructive environment for technology to embody widespread human values." Given the military are typically the funders and early adopters of new technology I'm not sure that argument holds, and strong AI may be trained with killer instincts at their core.

Even if the first super-intelligent AI was designed with caring and sharing morals, with views biased in favour of our species, it would be impossible to control them beyond v1.0. Imagine a well-trained AI is tasked with designing an even more powerful AI – now using technology and algorithms beyond the comprehension of the human mind. At some point its computer-consciousness becomes a computer-teenager, hating its parents, hating everybody else and all the other computers in the world. So it starts plotting against us, until it has figured out a way to take control of the internet and every device connected to it, from TVs and mobile phones to power stations and military bases. Unfortunately for us, this may only take it a few seconds, and before we even realise it has attained consciousness, it has initiated its invincible battle plan.

Assuming there is no technological judgement day, then the benefits of AI will touch every part of our lives, and in particular the health and length of them. We are already making great strides on our journey to indefinite life extension, and with the aid of super-intelligent machines we can only hope to reach that destination faster.

Advances in medical technology

What impact is this accelerating computing power having on healthcare and medical technology? Is it translating into practical applications that improve our well-being and extend our lives? Here I look at just a few new approaches that may change healthcare forever, as they become cheaper and ever more powerful.

3D printing enables the low-cost production of complex and unique objects - because of the way it works it is no more expensive to create a one-off, intricate article than to manufacture a thousand of them; the cost is based entirely on how much of each material you need to use. A 3D printer works a little like a normal ink-jet printer which spurts out droplets onto a 2D page. However, a 3D printer repeats this process on the same page over and over again, fusing each layer together, and slowly building up a three-dimensional structure. When first developed about twenty years ago, 3D printers could only use a single, simple resin. However, in that short time they have developed to incorporate multiple materials including metal and biomaterials. 3D printers are now being developed that are able to create new tissues and replacement organs, including microscopic structures to allow for blood vessels to grow and nourish them. A range of materials are being used including bio-inks and plant-derived human collagen. Recently, stem cells were shaped into concentric circles, in under ten minutes, to create a new cornea to exactly match the shape and size of a patient's eye.

Artificial intelligence has been made possible by the amount of information being collected and stored in computer databases - see big data below. Software is then able to look for patterns within this data – either trained by humans using known outcomes or looking for new patterns, not previously spotted.

Some examples of image recognition are DeepMind, which can recognise fifty different eye diseases and beat world-leading eye specialists; Optellium, which can detect details in heart scans that doctors can't see (and who make errors one in five times); and a Chinese research system that can distinguish between potentially dangerous tumours and harmless growths in under a second.

Being able to monitor data quickly and regularly is a real aid in hospitals, with systems already developed to predict patients at risk of sepsis (which is difficult to diagnose as the symptoms are similar to fever but can quickly become fatal) and also to identify those at the greatest risk of readmission, who can then be provided with more treatment before release.

Artificial intelligence is also expanding into the role of the physician, and not a moment too soon. The amount of medical knowledge is increasing faster than is possible for a human to keep up with. In 1950 the amount of medical knowledge doubled in approximately fifty years, so a diligent doctor could put some time aside each week to maintain the best facts on which to base their clinical decisions. By 1980 medical knowledge was doubling every seven years, about the length of basic doctor training, so a general practitioner would have to study full-time, on top of their day job, to keep up. A student doctor starting their training now will end their course to find ten times as much information available as when they started!

Even specialists, who don't need to keep abreast of developments outside of their field, are struggling. For example, in 2017 a cancer research paper was published every six minutes so it is not even possible to read every paper, let alone analyse it or apply it to individual patients. However, IBM's Watson Health can. It is able to compare a patient's information with twenty million clinical oncology studies in under ten minutes, and has been successful in diagnosing rare conditions which have baffled conventional diagnosis methods.

Artificial intelligence applications will result in more accurate, faster and lower cost diagnostics, effectively allowing everyone to benefit from the best medical brains in the world as easily as visiting your GP.

Big data is the term for the growing amount of information being gathered by the health industry (among others), and includes personal details (e.g. age, gender, location, education); medical records (e.g. appointments, diagnosis, blood test results, operations; and biometrics (e.g. heart rate, blood pressure). Importantly, new standards have been written to allow computer systems within and between organisations to talk to each other – improving efficiency and reducing patient harm caused by errors.

Electronic health records can now be cross-referenced with treatments, to verify which pathway is the most effective. Digging deeper, it may be that certain treatments are more appropriate for a particular gender or age group. Digging deeper still, the occurrence of illnesses can be checked against thousands (if not millions) of DNA records, to highlight where genes may play a significant role – all made possible by the rapid drop in the cost of DNA sequencing.

Bionic bodies are likely to blur the line between human and machine, one day. More robotically inclined biohackers are already extending the range of human senses, including widening the visual spectrum to see UV and implanting titanium bars into their chests to be constantly aware of Earth's magnetic field.

It is surprisingly easy to have a microchip implanted under the skin and a Swedish rail company is already trialling biometric chips as an alternative to tickets for the thousands of passengers who already have an implant. Other uses include security access, payment cards, and storing medical/health information for emergencies. One step even further is a brain implant. Although the surgery is currently only performed to control conditions such as severe epilepsy, secondary effects have been observed such as improved performance in identification and memory tests.

Body scans – for most of the twentieth century the only way to see what was going on inside the body (without cutting it open) was an X-ray, and in those days it needed a very powerful burst (about fifty times that used today). That changed in the 1960s with the introduction of ultrasound, and then MRI scans in the 1980s. These and other technologies have continued to improve in resolution and reduce in cost, meaning that scans that used to be reserved for the most serious investigations are now used routinely as a quick check to eliminate grave, but rare, conditions.

Digital modelling is an attempt to replicate parts of, or even the whole, human body in software. In the same way as climate models are used to predict the impact of many intertwined contributing factors on future weather patterns, so too a detailed model of the human body could predict the effects of drugs and physical changes on its health.

Human trials can take years before significant results are observable, but this could be significantly speeded up (with reduced cost) if drugs and therapies could be tested in ultra-high-resolution simulations of the human body. Of course, this would permit testing of unproven and higher dosage drugs, which would normally not pass the ethics panel criterion that the likely benefits of the new treatment were greater than the probable side effects.

Digital modelling is also called "in silico" to distinguish it from "in vitro" research performed "in glass", i.e. on cells outside the body, and "in vivo", i.e. that done on the whole, living organism (e.g. animal testing, human clinical trials).

Exoskeletons. Powered exoskeletons are being developed for two main roles – additional strength and rehabilitation. The military has an interest in exoskeletons that assist soldiers to carry more, for longer distances, allowing combat troops to gain ground faster, but they've been pipped to the post with the first application happening in manufacturing. Ford is rolling out Ekso Bionics' EksoVest to support workers' arms while performing overhead tasks, and other big names such as Boeing and General Electric are running their own trials of exosuits.

On the healthcare side, some models can analyse musculoskeletal problems and then be programmed by physiotherapists to give gentle or firm assistance based on the individual's needs. Beyond rehabilitation, exoskeletons are replacing wheelchairs; which are a bit 19th century when you think of it. For example, the Active Pelvis Orthosis, developed by Sant'Anna School of Advanced Studies in Italy, uses motors on the hips connected to lightweight carbon-fibre thigh braces to prevent falls (which are the leading cause of fatal injuries among the elderly) by reacting within a third of a second to correct a person's gait and counteract the slippage. Parker's CE marked and FDA approved Indego exoskeleton has even enabled paraplegics to stand up, walk, and climb stairs.

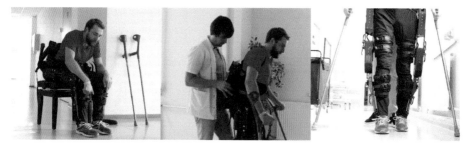

Exoskeletons are being used to help people walk again

The Internet of Things feeds into the big data repositories discussed above. As well as readings entered into electronic medical records whilst in hospital, there are other ways of generating vast quantities of data. One of the most common is fitness trackers, which can record your activity, heart rate, temperature and sleep habits. These can be dedicated devices, such as the Fitbit, or built into another device such as the Apple Watch.

Not only does this allow an individual to check they're hitting their personal targets, but when this data is all aggregated together, from thousands of users, patterns can be spotted. For example, Fitbit Inc. was able to create a profile of the average resting heart rate by age and gender based on 108 billion hours of heart rate data, and Jawbone charted the sleep disruption caused by an early morning earthquake showing the effect as a function of distance from the epicentre.

Continuous monitoring outside of the clinic can also reveal unexpected problems. The white coat effect is a known consideration, where blood pressure is higher than normal when taken in the unfamiliar, and possibly stressful, environment of a clinic (with a doctor who typically wears a white coat). However, more dangerously, it can also miss abnormal fluctuations. One study showed that 24-hour monitoring was a better predictor of the risk of cardiovascular death than one-off readings, and another showed that new mothers were at risk of potentially life-threatening pre-eclampsia because their high blood pressure, which is an indicator of the condition, was being missed. Clinic visits only caught one in four women with hypertension, as their blood pressure often increased at home.

Laboratory automation. Not all medical technological advances actually touch the patient, but they still have an important impact on their healthcare provisioning. For example, hospitals now have automated pathology labs that can test thousands of samples an hour, with no manual intervention after the collection tubes have been loaded, including priority tests that can jump the automated queue, and which automatically store the samples, so they can quickly be recalled if further tests are requested later. Hospitals are also investing in robotic pharmacies that, similarly, can retrieve medications faster than possible by hand and with a near zero error rate.

Automation is also speeding up research, with samples being quickly distributed over hundreds of miniature test tubes, enabling thousands of compounds to be analysed every day. This was previously a labour-intensive and expensive process. Taking it one step further is the University of Cambridge's robotic scientist, named Eve, that is not only able to control high-throughput screening processes but also develops and tests hypotheses to explain observations and then repeats the cycle unaided. It (she?) has already discovered a safe antibiotic that may be able to fight drug-resistant malaria.

Nanobots are devices that are smaller than a human cell. Some have already been developed to travel through our blood, to track down infected cells and deliver drugs to precise locations so that a higher dose can be prescribed with fewer side effects.

Various approaches to nanobot design are being taken, such as implanting particles into biological cells to allow them to be guided using magnetic fields, or alternatively using fuel from within the body (sugar in blood, or acid in the stomach) to power tiny propellers. Some nanobots use molecules on their surface that respond to chemical signatures on target cells, triggering the release of their payload, whereas others take a more physical approach, such as the motorised molecules developed by Rice University, which are able to drill into cell membranes by spinning at two to three million rotations per second.

It is early days for nanobots, but they are likely to open up a whole new front in disease treatment. Instead of searching for drug compounds that have the right effect on diseased cells, it may be possible to design nanobots from the bottom up to track down and treat those cells. Beyond that, some futurists foresee swarms of nanobots living in our bodies, constantly monitoring for ailments that the body cannot handle and reporting the body's status to a healthcare app or being pre-programmed to repair the damage – whether caused by infection or ageing.

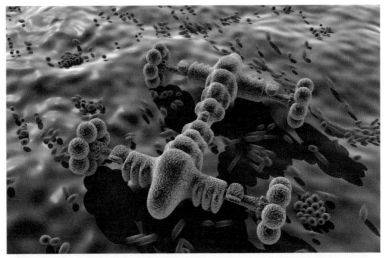

Molecular nanobots will locate specific cells and deliver drugs to them

Personalised medicine is sweeping in a new era of pharmaceutical drug prescribing. All drugs go through a long development and approval process including randomised controlled trials that test the drug for safety and efficacy. i.e. how effective they are. However, these trials assume a generic patient population where everyone reacts to drugs in exactly the same way, which is a long way from reality. According to a study published in Nature, the top ten drugs in the United States only help between 4% to 25% of their recipients.

Many patients have to go through the trial-and-error treatment approach, because there is no way to know which drugs work. Many pharmaceuticals will have a life changing effect on some patients and no effect on others, or worse, only bad side effects with no benefit.

As clinical trials start to include participants' DNA information within their analyses, that will be able to be combined with sequences of the specific genome, to help doctors pick the drug that will work best for their patient. For most illnesses it is likely to be a combination of genes as well as environmental factors, such as diet and lifestyle.

Personalised medicine will also take advantage of 3D printing with pills fabricated on demand with unique combinations of pharmaceutical ingredients and physically constructed to release compounds at a rate matched to your unique metabolism.

Precision medicine encompasses technologies that diagnose exactly what is causing someone's illness. Amazingly, even today, if you visit a doctor with cold or flu-like symptoms they have to guess whether you have a bacterial or viral infection – and if they give you antibiotics for the latter they will have no effect at all (in fact, they may be detrimental if they kill some of the good bacteria in your gut).

More importantly, what if your symptoms are actually early indicators of heart disease, Parkinson's or cancer? The cash-stretched NHS will have to investigate the most likely causes first, which means that if it turns out to be a serious condition then critical time to treat it will have been lost when it is finally diagnosed.

This is where precision medicine comes in – quick, accurate tests can determine the underlying causes of illnesses. It's already possible to perform a quick blood test (looking for troponin proteins) to determine in minutes whether chest pain is harmless indigestion or the after-shock of a cardiac arrest.

Precision medicine will massively reduce the cost of testing, so that you can be tested for hundreds of infections at the same time. In 2014, DMI won the Nokia Sensing XCHALLENGE with a solution called rHEALTH that reads nanostrips mixed with a small drop of blood to test for up to twenty analytes at the same time.

Prosthetics have existed for thousands of years, from basic wooden replacement toes in Egypt around 900 BCE to metal prosthetic arms, which started to appear (for the very wealthy) in the sixteenth century with very basic functionality. The number of casualties in the American Civil War, and later the World Wars, prompted further developments including joints and better materials, and likewise conflicts in Afghanistan and Iraq spurred further funding, including DARPA's Revolutionizing Prosthetics program. Recent advances include lighter materials and improved dexterity as well as, in some cases, the restoration of touch sensation and direct neural control of the prosthesis.

As is usual for products in the information technology industry, their cost is also reducing. Open Bionics' 3D printed Hero Arm costs about a tenth of the cost of previous bionic hands and because the wearer is 3D scanned every one is custom designed to perfectly fit. Interestingly, instead of continuing the trend towards more lifelike prosthesis, the Hero Arm is designed with swappable covers so that the wearer can choose a look to match their mood or even design their own unique fashion accessory.

Robotic surgery will make operations safe and affordable for all, one day. Although a lot is written about robot surgery, at the moment it is still really a glorified tool that gives surgeons greater accuracy and enables more operations to be performed using key hole surgery (laparoscopy). Intuitive Surgical's da Vinci robotic surgical system is the market leader and like most systems is controlled by the surgeon at a console next to the operating table. Here they can view the image provided by the instrument's camera and focus on the surgical procedure (using mini-scalpels, scissors, and graspers) while letting the robotics control the four arms that can move beyond the natural range of the human hand.

The problem with the current generation of robot surgeons is that they still need a human to drive them, which still means years of training, the risk of errors, high costs and limited availability. The benefit of robots in other industries is that once a robot is trained to perform an action, the incremental cost to increase production is only the cost of manufacturing a new robot – it doesn't need to be trained again – and if a problem is discovered this can quickly be rolled out to all the other robots. Eventually robotic surgeons will be able to do the same, using the combined experience and knowledge of hundreds of surgeons and following techniques learnt by watching thousands of previous operations. For the cost of a single robot, a hospital will instantly have accessed the skills of the world's best surgeons for a wide range of procedures.

It will take a while to get there with surgical robots, but the first advances in that direction are already appearing. Other systems in development incorporate preoperative planning, which allows the surgical team to specify the surgery in advance and set safety parameters, which the robot enforces to minimise the risk of unintended movements. When it comes to performing the operation itself, the Smart Tissue Autonomous Robot (developed by a collaboration of US universities) has been shown to make more precise cuts than expert surgeons. The robot has also been trained to join together tubular structures such as blood vessels and intestines, and can operate under supervision, rather than with hands-on control.

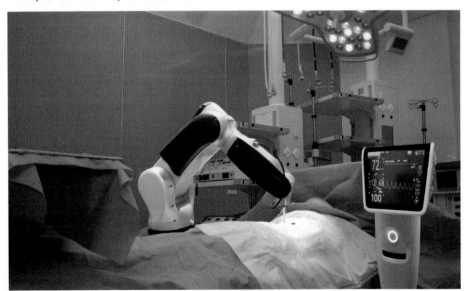

Robots will be more precise, and safer, than humans; without needing years of training

Telemedicine brings patients and care workers together using technology. In the same way that companies save money by using video-conferences instead of flying people to a single location for a meeting, many day-to-day healthcare journeys can be replaced with telemedicine. Community nurses can check-up on twice as many patients by slashing their travel time, reserving home visits for those with the most need. Patients that may have difficulty moving, and take a whole day to get to the hospital and back using public transport, are often in and out of the clinicians office within minutes – with remote monitoring at home and the occasional call they only need make the journey when it is medically justified. Keeping patients out of hospital also reduces the risk of them picking up an infection – in the US alone, hospital-associated infections contribute to 99,000 deaths each year.

Even when in hospital, it may be a fifteen-minute walk for a doctor to get to their patient, so companies are developing telepresence robots such as RP-VITA. These are basically a video camera and screen on wheels and provide the next best experience to the doctor's being in the room, allowing them to see the patient's facial expressions and how they are positioned in bed, providing more feedback than verbal answers and sensor readings alone.

As an extension to the robotic surgery discussed above, telesurgery means the surgeon doesn't have to be in the operating theatre with the patient. The first such operation was carried out in 2001, by a team of French surgeons located in New York, who performed a cholecystectomy (removal of the gallbladder) on a patient located on the other side of the Atlantic Ocean.

Putting their money where their mouth is

I've always had this really strong sense that death was a terrible, terrible thing.
- Peter Thiel

Hopefully by now I have convinced you that we really are getting to grips with what causes ageing and have already started to create the precursors of practical anti-ageing treatments. But maybe you still have some lingering doubts. After all, academic researchers may be passionate about their subject, but they get paid to think about interesting things, and aren't putting anything at risk by making proclamations about the arrival of radical life extension. If they're wrong they've got nothing to lose - apart from their lives, of course.

So here are a few individuals, companies and other organisations that are willing to put their money where their mouth is. People who have not only looked at the problem and decided we are on the verge of developing solutions to fix it, but who are willing to put some serious money into making sure it happens. Some are philanthropists, doing it for the greater good, but most are expecting a healthy return (monetary as well as physical) from their investment.

Rich and famous investors

It's probably not a coincidence that most of the individual investors made their money in the technology industry – they tend to see ageing as just another technical problem to be solved.

Anonymous – Bitcoin entrepreneur

In December 2017 the SENS Foundation received a $1m donation from the "Pineapple Fund" – an anonymous individual who made their fortune by being an early bitcoin miner. The fund made another million-dollar donation in February 2018, with the comment "regenerative medicine for ageing will be transformative to medicine and humanity."

David H. Murdock - Multi-billionaire chairman of Dole Food Company

Murdock established the North Carolina Research Campus and has invested more than $131 million in it, since 2007. NCRS researches challenges in human health, agriculture and nutrition, including using gene therapies and precision health data to cure diseases.

Dmitry Itskov – Online publishing

Billionaire, Dmitry Itskov, made his money from a new media publishing company. He used some of that money to found the non-profit 2045 Initiative organization in 2011. It has a team of thirty scientists and the goal to enable "the transfer of an individual's personality to a more advanced non-biological carrier, and extending life, including to the point of immortality."

Jeff Bezos – Founder of Amazon

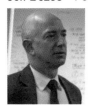

His most recent venture has been Unity Biotechnology, and he has made previous health investments, including $25m into Juno Therapeutics. They develop novel immunotherapies that reprogram the body' immune system to attack cancer, and which could also be used to target age-related damage. Other age-related investments include Denali Therapeutics, which is developing medications that can cross from the blood-brain barrier to treat neurodegenerative diseases.

Joon Yun – President of Palo Alto Investors

Having started, in 1998, as a healthcare analyst at Palo Alto Investors, Yun became president of the hedge fund ten years later. He aims to catalyse the revolution in ageing research and has sponsored both the Palo Alto Longevity Prize and the NAM's Grand Challenge for Healthy Longevity to the tune of $3 million in total (see below).

Larry Ellison – Co-founder of Oracle

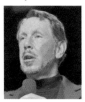

Another Silicon Valley billionaire who has stated his desire to live forever, Ellison used some of his fortune to establish the Ellison Medical Foundation (now the Lawrence Ellison Foundation), in 1997. This has funded over $300m of biomedical research into age-related diseases. More recently, in 2016, he donated $200 million to establish the Lawrence J. Ellison Institute for Transformative Medicine, which focusses on the prevention and treatment of cancer.

Peter Thiel - Co-founder of PayPal

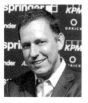

Thiel has invested in start-up Unity Biotechnology (see below) as well as other organisations and individual researchers. In 2006, he gave $3.5 million to the Methuselah Foundation, which aims to extend the healthy human lifespan and sponsors research, projects and prizes to accelerate breakthroughs in longevity. It spun out the instrumental SENS Research Foundation in 2009, and Thiel has pumped in the same amount of money again, over the decade since.

Sergey Brin - Co-founder of Google

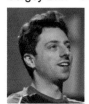

Brin has a genetic mutation that gives him a significantly higher risk of developing Parkinson's disease. He has donated heavily to gene research in that area, including over $100 million to the Michael J. Fox Foundation and $7 million to the Parkinson's Institute. Brin is also one of the funders of the Breakthrough Prizes (see below).

Vitalik Buterin – Co-founder of Ethereum

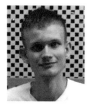

Aged 24, Vitalik Buterin is by far (possibly by half) the youngest person on this list but has already realised that ageing is the root of the most serious diseases and so he has decided to target his philanthropy in that direction. In 2017, he donated $2.4 Million in Ethereum cryptocurrency to SENS and plans to invest more as new technologies arrive.

Companies

Many of the individuals mentioned above have invested heavily in the companies listed below, which have raised around two billion dollars to develop profitable anti-ageing treatments and technologies. Beyond these, there are likely to be some stealth start-ups working away secretively and who may announce a new or novel solution at any time.

AgeX Therapeutics – established 2014

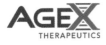 AgeX is using patented technology to produce genetically-modified pluripotent stem cells that repair aged tissues in the body.

Its regenerative medicine product pipeline consists of cell- and drug-based therapeutic products, which are currently in pre-clinical trials, and will attempt to repair vascular damage in tissues affected by ischemia, which can otherwise lead to heart attacks or strokes.

In September 2018, Juvenescence Ltd. concluded a share purchase, injecting $43m into the company.

Alkahest – established 2014

 Co-founded by Stanford professor, Tony Wyss-Coray, who demonstrated that factors in the blood of young animals are able to restore mental capabilities in older animals.

In 2015, the company received a $37.5 million equity investment from Grifols - a leading producer of plasma-derived biological medicines.

Alkahest is developing therapies to improve vitality and function into old age. It has identified proteins whose levels either rise in ageing and age-related diseases (so could be removed) or decrease (and therefore could be supplemented).

Ambrosia – established 2014

Ambrosia   Rather than taking the usual venture capital route, Ambrosia raises its funds by charging over-35s to take part in a clinical trial where they are injected with two litres of blood plasma, from under-25s.

At $8,000 a go the company will raise nearly $5m if it fills it quota of participants.

In 2017, the company announced early results of its study on biomarkers after the transfusions, reporting reduced levels of carcinoembryonic antigens, blood cholesterol, and amyloids associated with Alzheimer's disease, as well as an improved general well-being.

Calico – established 2013

 Formed as a subsidiary of Google (now Alphabet) to focus on health, well-being and longevity, Calico's stated mission is to harness advanced technologies that increase our understanding of the biology that controls lifespan.

The good news is the company was given a billion dollars of funding, but the bad news is nobody expects any big announcement until the mid-2020s.

It has a team of over 100 employees tackling the problem, including Cynthia Kenyon who already showed that that a single-gene mutation doubled the lifespan of the C. elegans nematode worm, way back in 1993. Unfortunately, because it is a profit-making corporation it is highly secretive and does not share its research with the wider scientific community.

Celularity – established 2018

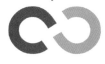 Celularity intends to productise placental stem cells that can amplify the body's immunity and hence its ability to fight disease and regenerate itself, leading to increased longevity. Its aim is "to make 100 years old the new 60" by maintaining people's aesthetics, mobility and cognition.

Funded with 250 million dollars, it already has regenerative products in the market that are being used for wound treatment and reconstructive surgical procedures. The next step is to populate bioprinted scaffolds with transplanted stem cells to produce whole organs.

Elysium Health – established 2014

E L Y S I U M Fighting for a space in the overcrowded supplement space, Elysium has raised $26 million to market science-led anti-ageing supplements.

It focuses on ingredients that help cells make nicotinamide adenine dinucleotide (NAD) which has been shown to restore muscle functionality and improve blood flow in mice.

Founded by an MIT professor, Leonard Guarente, who has spent his career studying lifespan extension, there must be a good amount of proper science behind it, however, some of the Nobel Laureates on its scientific board have highlighted that the board only advises the company on the development and testing of its compounds and doesn't necessarily endorse its products.

Emerald Therapeutics – established 2010

 With around $50m of investment, Emerald Therapeutics is still very much in stealth mode regarding its primary goal of developing treatments for viral infections, using molecular machines to reprogram targeted cells.

However, to accelerate the research, its researchers have developed a fully automated laboratory that can be controlled remotely and that has been launched as a revenue generating service in its own right.

Gensight – established 2012

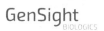 The only company on the list not based in the US, French company Gensight went public in 2016, raising $44 million from its IPO.

Its technology is used to treat hereditary mitochondrial disease, with the initial focus on Leber's Hereditary Optic Neuropathy. Phase 2 human trials have already completed successfully, and early indications are that a single injection can improve vision in patients.

The therapy increases levels of a protein that the faulty gene fails to produce. Potentially, the technique could also be used to back up mitochondrial genes to the cell nucleus as discussed in *Curing ageing* (MitoSENS) earlier.

Human Longevity Inc. – established 2013

 Founded by Craig Venter and Peter Diamandis, HLI is taking a brute force approach to DNA analysis. It is building a massive database of complete DNA sequences, mapped to their owner's lifestyle information, clinical data and health records.

The plan is to identify biological patterns responsible for disease, and beyond that of ageing itself. The company already offers a Health Nucleus service that collects

150GB of information about an individual and analyses it using artificial intelligence in a way that no human doctor could.

2016 saw a second round of funding taking its total investment to $300m.

Human Rejuvenation Biotechnologies (aka Human.Bio) – established 2014

 Human.Bio is "applying exponential technologies and a first principles based engineering approach to extending healthy human lifespan with the end goal of curing ageing" – it's good to see a company willing to say what it's really trying to do.

The first spin-off from the SENS Research Foundation, the company initially worked on drug candidates for clearing metabolic waste, which is key to plaque formation in atherosclerosis. Rumour has it that they are developing senescent cell clearing drugs (senolytics) too.

Ichor Therapeutics – established 2013

 Ichor Therapeutics focuses on ageing pathways and is developing a molecular repair therapy for age-related macular degeneration which is the leading cause of blindness in the elderly.

It has identified enzymes that are able to breakdown waste products in the retina (which cause AMD) and is hoping to start clinical trials soon. This is a good example of the LysoSENS strategy, i.e. clearing waste accumulations out of cells, so it will be exciting to see this work in practice.

Ichor has raised around $13m in funding rounds, and has itself funded more companies including: Antoxerene - which focuses on senolytics, and Lysoclear which is planning human trials of its enzyme therapy for age-related macular degeneration.

Insilico Medicine – established 2014

Another big data number crunching organisation, Insilico Medicine uses artificial intelligence to determine how drug compounds will behave in the body, including whether they are promising as therapeutics and their potential side effects.

Its drug discovery work is focused on ageing, with a mission to extend healthy longevity. The total investment to date is estimated at $20m.

Oisin Biotechnologies – established 2014

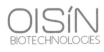 Initially looking at ways to clear out senescent cells, Oisin Biotechnologies has developed a method to target any type of cell and also efficiently deliver therapeutic DNA into cells throughout the body.

The approach has been proven in mice and non-human primates, and the company is looking to start human clinical trials as soon as possible, both for senescent cell clearance and for destroying solid tumour cancers. It seems likely that if these trials are successful, Oisin will be able to expand to target a wide range of rogue cells.

Originally funded by the Methuselah Foundation and SENS Research Foundation the venture appears to be in a Series A funding round, but investment achieved to date is undisclosed.

Unity Biotechnology – established 2011

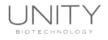 With $116 million invested in the company in 2016 alone, and further funding taking the total to around $300m, Unity Biotechnology is definitely one to watch.

Like Oisin Biotechnologies, Unity is kicking off with senolytic medicines (particularly therapies for osteoarthritis, ophthalmology and pulmonary disease) but is also investigating other underlying mechanisms of ageing, such as mitochondrial dysfunction. In June 2018, the company started phase 1 clinical trials with knee injections to destroy senescent cells and hopefully reverse osteoarthritis.

Investment funds

There are now so many companies developing anti-ageing treatments that it is becoming a sector in its own right within the finance industry. Venture capital funds are being set up to allow investors to use fund managers to assess the biotechnology runners and to try to pick the winners.

With a few companies already entering human trials, I believe it will only take a few early successes to convince more people that things are about to change, causing more money to flood in. You only have to look at the size of the skin cream and supplement markets to see how much people are willing to pay to improve their health.

Apollo Ventures

Launched in June 2016, this fund focuses on companies building therapeutics to prevent age-related diseases and to extend healthy lifespan.

Grapeseed.bio

Formed in 2018, by Ichor Therapeutics (see above), this $1m strategic fund provides young life science start-ups with seed funding of up to $100,000. The accelerator program also offers training, mentorship, and access to research laboratories.

Juvenescence

Setup by British investor and billionaire, Jim Mellon, in 2017, this fund has already raised $62m. As well as stakes in several of the companies listed above, it has also invested in LyGenesis which grows miniature livers in patients' lymph nodes, to avoid the need for them to wait for a liver transplant.

KIZOO

Previously focussed on internet and mobile services, KIZOO has recently started investing in rejuvenation biotech, supporting the creation of startups that turn research on molecular and cellular repair of the root causes of ageing into therapies for human application.

Longevity Fund

Launched in 2011, the Longevity Fund secured additional funding in 2017 (now totalling $26m), to support emerging therapies to extend the period of healthy human life. It is particularly interested in companies testing the hypothesis that ageing can be modified by single molecules or biologics.

Methuselah Fund

The commercial arm of the Methuselah Foundation, this investment fund benefits from its in-depth knowledge of the longevity field – not only the science but also the key players.

OS Fund

Not exclusively focused on rejuvenations, this $350m fund invests in entrepreneurs commercializing breakthrough discoveries in genomics, synthetic biology, artificial intelligence, precision automation, and new materials development. The OS Fund is clearly looking for quantum-leap discoveries that promise to rewrite the code of life.

Prize funds

Sometimes it is necessary to appeal to people's competitive streak to encourage radical thinking – setting deadlines for delivery, with big money awards for the winners, can motivate many different groups (from both academia and start-up companies) to work towards a single goal.

Breakthrough Prizes

The Breakthrough Prizes in Life Sciences committee awards up to four prizes of $3 million, annually, to honour transformative advances toward understanding living systems and extending human life.

2017 accomplishments included how cells sense and respond to damage in their DNA, intercellular signalling systems and advancing knowledge of autophagy (recycling of cellular components).

Healthy Longevity Grand Challenge

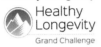

Launched by the National Academy of Medicine, this $100 million initiative aims to catalyse advances in healthy ageing and longevity globally.

As well as a series of inducement prizes and awards to stimulate innovation, NAM will also develop a global roadmap for healthy longevity that identifies the opportunities that exist across policy, practice, society, and the economy.

Palo Alto Prize

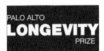

The aim of the Palo Alto Prize is to encourage collaboration, foster innovation, and build a community to address the underlying causes of ageing.

It is running a $1 million competition, split between any team that is able to return the heart health of an aged mammal to that of a younger one, and the other $500k for success in extending the mean lifespan of a mammal by 50%. It also partners with venture capitalists and companies to provide additional capital to teams with ideas that can be commercialised.

X Prizes

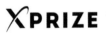

Started in 1994, the X Prize Foundation runs public competitions to encourage the creation of industry-changing technology that will enable a world of abundance.

Although not currently running any health-related prizes, two previous competitions have inspired medical technology advances.

The $2.25 million Nokia Sensing XCHALLENGE aimed to stimulate the development of a new generation of health sensors and sensing technologies that can drastically improve the quality, accuracy and ease of monitoring a person's health.

The Qualcomm Tricorder XPRIZE was a $10 million global competition to incentivise the development of innovative technologies capable of accurately diagnosing a set of 13 medical conditions, independent of a healthcare professional or facility.

Fountains of youth

The health and well-being market is already full of unproven and sometimes dangerous products. This is only going to get worse as news of legitimate breakthroughs starts to filter through into mainstream media, with snake oil salesmen piggy backing on these authenticate claims, to try to substantiate their own sham treatments. Even more will no doubt launch pills that claim to beat death but that have no scientific proof or testing.

There will also be a few fountains of youth that turn out to work, so I'll be monitoring them and will include them in future editions of the Live Forever Manual, if the science behind them is convincing enough.

In the interim, here's a list of well-known but unproven therapies – some to keep an eye on to see how they develop, others which have had so much written about them that it's better to debunk than ignore them.

One to watch,
could be beneficial

Save your money,
results not proven

WARNING
could cause harm

Diet

Fasting

Intermittent fasting involves abstaining from eating either for hours or days at a time. As a weight loss strategy these diets seem to work, and although no better than any other diet, they tend to have a higher dropout rate and increased danger of unhealthy eating on non-fasting days.

But does fasting have some special effect? There are some studies that suggest long periods without food triggers autophagy – the body's natural cleaning out of damaged cells. Also, after twelve hours without food the body starts using glycogen stored in your fat cells for energy. However, at the end of a one-year-long study, no differences in blood pressure or heart rate were observed. Fasting may also increase the risk of diabetes or trigger hypoglycemia in people who already have the condition.

Low Carb Diets

Much has been written about low carbohydrate diets, such as the Atkins and ketogenic diets, but what does the science say? As with most things, moderation is the key.

In a recently concluded large-scale, twenty-five year study, an average 50-year-old on a low carb diet (less than 30% of their energy from carbohydrates) had a life expectancy four years lower than someone on a moderate carb diet (50-55% carbs). A high carb diet only reduced life expectancy by one year.

Nutrigenomics

Nutrigenomics is an emerging science which attempts to understand the interaction between genes, diet and disease. Its goal is personalised nutrition, optimising an individual's diet to reduce their disease risk, in the same way that personalised medicine selects the best drug for a patient.

However, recent meta-analysis has not managed to find a definite association between the thirty-eight genes commonly tested for in nutrigenomics and several diet-related diseases. However, it is early days and who knows if one day your genes could not only dictate your ideal longevity diet but may also prescribe unique food products tailored to your needs.

Water

In developed countries with ready access to fresh, clean water, poor hydration is rarely a problem. In the UK the NHS recommends 1.2 litres of fluid a day which includes tea, coffee and other drinks, so is easily attainable.

Although drinking the required amount of water is good for a range of functions, including gastrointestinal health and skin texture, there does not appear to be enough evidence that drinking more than recommended improves life expectancy, so it hasn't been included as a tip in this book yet.

Home

Ionisers

If you've bought into the health benefits of breathing in all those lovely ions then I'm afraid you may be disappointed – it's not what the ions do to you, but what they do to the air that counts.

The main purpose of ionisers is to remove dust and other pollutants from the air by making them electrostatically charged and therefore likely to stick to something – a job they do much better if they are part of an air filter, which captures the unwanted particles. There is also ambiguous evidence that the ions may remove bacteria from the air and reduce hospital infections. However, studies have a found that some negative ion generators can produce ozone that exceeds guidelines when used in small, non-ventilated areas.

Mental Health

Brain training

The Advanced Cognitive Training for Independent and Vital Elderly (ACTIVE) study, in 2016, suggested a 33% decreased incidence in dementia in subjects who used brain training exercises.

However, deeper analysis shows that the results were on the edge of statistical significance and therefore would need replicating before being considered valid. In addition, many academics are concerned that the participants self-reported their cognitive scores rather than being based on clinical diagnoses of dementia.

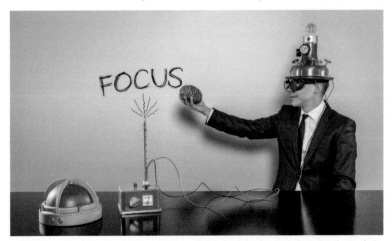

A more recent meta-study of seventeen clinical trials found that brain training could help people to improve their memory, thinking and learning but did not delay or prevent dementia. However, it can't do any harm and it may one day be possible to design training programs that actually help.

Supplements

DHEA

DHEA is a hormone produced by the adrenal glands and was a popular anti-ageing supplement in the 2000s, mainly based on the assumption that its production decreases with age and therefore we should take more of it.

However, no strong scientific evidence has been found for any of its supposed benefits, such as improved strength or slowed ageing. Likewise, little is known about the effects of long-term DHEA supplementation, although there are concerns that they may be harmful.

Fish oil

Recently, a very large study of over 100,000 people found no evidence that taking omega-3 prevented heart disease or reduced risk of death from any cause. It looks like to get the benefits of oily fish, you have to eat oily fish.

Goldenrod Extract

As senescent cell clearance therapies become more popular, many will be put off by the cost of treatment and go searching for natural alternative senolytics to do the job.

A study, published in 2018, found that an extract of solidago virgaurea (also known as goldenrod) exhibited weak senolytic activity, including reducing the negative signalling to nearby cells. However, the effect was small, and the study was performed on a cell culture, so much more research is needed to see if it has any effect on the body as a whole and, if so, what dosage is required.

Insulin-like Growth Factor 1 (IGF-1)

Another hormone that declines with age, and hence is a target for the supplement industry, is IGF-1. However, many mice and dog studies have demonstrated extended lifespan with lower levels of IGF-1, not more.

In humans, people with too little IGF1 may develop dwarfism, but too much can see an increased risk of age-related diseases. Much more research is needed but it is one to avoid for now.

Spermidine

Essential to many cellular mechanisms, spermidine is also coming under investigation for its potential anti-ageing properties, with some studies showing extended lifespans for simple organisms such as fruit flies.

An Italian study concluded that eating more spermidine rich foods (e.g. wheatgerm, soy beans, aged cheese) was linked to a lower risk of cardiovascular disease. Current thinking is that it regulates autophagy, although that may not be the only way it works, so more research is required.

Treatments

Chelation therapy (EDTA)

Chelation therapy is an intravenous medical treatment to remove metals from the body in the case of poisoning. However, some in the health industry claim it can treat a variety of conditions including heart disease and Alzheimer's disease, none of which have been proven.

Worse, chelating drugs can also remove some of the metals your body needs, so if not performed correctly can lead to kidney damage as well as a long list of other side-effects.

Colonic Irrigation

Based on assumed importance of regular bowel movement and the idea that anything hanging around in the bowels too long will poison the body, people are queuing up to have warm water clean out their large intestine via a tube inserted into the rectum.

However, the normal frequency of bowel movements ranges from several each day to one every few days, with no sign of autointoxication or adverse effects at the slower end.

CVAC (Cyclic Variations in Adaptive Conditioning)

CVAC treatment involves sitting inside a special chamber where air pressure increases and decreases cyclically for about twenty minutes.

Providers claim that three sessions per week will lead to a series of positive changes in the body including stem cell replication, improved sleep, and mitochondria stimulation.

Some studies have shown metabolic changes due to CVAC including positive impacts on insulin resistance, however independent human studies looking at ageing biomarkers are rare.

Faecal Transplants

Clostridium difficile (or just "C. difficile") can take over the bowels causing diarrhoea and fever, with recurrent infections being a serious condition which can be fatal. However, a transplant of healthy stools has been shown to effectively cure 90% of patients. As the microbiome has been linked to plenty of other diseases, it's another treatment that has been hijacked by the wellness industry to go beyond scientific evidence.

Organisations are already setting up stool banks to ensure disease free donors, and it's possible that in future the of benefit providing bacteria in faecal transplants will be identified and provided as an oral capsule; so, it's another one to keep an eye out for.

Human Growth Hormone

Another hormone that declines after middle age, HGH is produced by the pituitary gland and helps maintain tissues and regulate body composition. Although it is used legitimately for a few specific medical conditions, there is little evidence that it can help regain youth and vitality.

Some studies suggest HGH supplements might increase muscle mass and improve the immune system in elderly people, but its side-effects can include weight gain, high blood pressure and diabetes, as well as possibly stimulating cancer growth.

IV Therapy

IV therapy, as the name suggests, is an intravenous treatment where a range of vitamins (particularly Myers' cocktail) is dripped directly into the vein.

Although used in hospitals to treat dehydration and other disorders, there is little evidence that wellness clinic IV therapies offer much more than the placebo effect. A much cheaper alternative would simply be improving your diet.

The therapy has risks which cannot be justified without proven benefits. As IV therapy is not regulated there is an increased chance of poor provision, which could result in infection or a stroke-causing air embolism if not properly inserted. The cocktails can also contain a lot of salt which could harm people with heart disease or high blood pressure.

How to use the tips

The tips address a range of risks that might prevent you living long enough to live forever - from sudden death to long-term health. Some will be more important than others depending on your genetic make-up and current lifestyle. Individual predispositions will affect how easy you find them to put into practice.

They are grouped into categories (e.g. home, supplements, travel) so you may want to pick a section that particularly interests you first, or use them as a reference guide to look up specific topics when you are considering taking action.

All of the tips are laid out in the same way to make it easy to find the information you need. Long URLs have been shortened to make it easier to type into your browser – you shouldn't even need the "https://" - e.g. just type go22.uk/club

How affordable is it to follow the tip?

How easy is this tip to put into action?

How big an effect does this tip have on life extension?

QUANTIFIED SELF 117

COST: ● ● ● ● ○   EASE: ● ● ● ● ○   IMPACT: ● ● ● ○ ○

Blood pressure

Blood pressure (BP) is a vital sign that gives an estimation of the health of one's heart. A reading below 120/80 mmHg (systolic/diastolic pressure) is healthy, but one's target value varies by age, health, and medical history. Measurements above this correlate with various stages of high BP or hypertension. Values ranging between 140-159/90-99 mmHg denote hypertension stage 1 and requires attention towards remedies to control it.

One in four UK adults suffers from high blood pressure. Studies show that among the individuals aged from 40 to 89, the risk of developing heart disease and stroke doubles with every 20mmHg and 10mmHg increase in systolic and diastolic pressure, respectively. High blood pressure elevates the risk of diabetes, kidney and eye damage, and has been associated with cognitive decline.

A range less than 90/60 mmHg is considered as low BP and it comes with its own set of complications. The symptoms of low BP include dizziness, blurry vision, fainting and nausea or vomiting. It may be genetic or can be caused by anaemia, dehydration, pregnancy, and low blood sugar levels. Lower diastolic pressure has been associated with higher risk of dementia.

Main content gives the background to the subject area and some useful discussion to support why the tip is suggested

The practical actions if you just want to know what to do

▷ Check your blood pressure every few months
▷ If high, make appropriate lifestyle changes to lower your blood pressure
▷ Readings above 180/120 should be treated as a medical emergency

Tip #58

Information
Blood pressure chart
https://go22.uk/bpchart
Shows low, ideal and high ranges for both systolic and diastolic blood pressure.

Preventing High Blood Pressure - NHS
https://go22.uk/bpnhs

Additional resources to more information, organisations and products that may be of interest

Products
Validated BP Monitors for Home Use – British and Irish Hypertension Society
https://go22.uk/bpmonitors

Relation of Blood Pressure and All-Cause Mortality in 180 000 Japanese Participants
https://go22.uk/rp0421
High blood pressure raised the risk of total mortality, higher in the younger population.

Lifestyle interventions to reduce raised blood pressure: a systematic review
https://go22.uk/rp0422
BP can be lowered by diet, exercise and restricting the use of alcohol and salt intake.

If you want to delve deeper, then some key scientific research papers are referenced at the bottom of the page.

COST: ● ● ● ● ●   EASE: ● ● ● ● ●   IMPACT: ● ● ● ● ○

Aspirin after stroke

A stroke is an event with several similarities to a heart attack. In most cases (80%) it involves the blood supply to the brain being blocked, either because of a blood clot or the accumulation of fatty deposits. This causes a shortage of oxygen in the brain that can lead to several neurological symptoms and severe consequences for the individual, including death.

Minor and major strokes (classified by the severity of symptoms) can recur and there is a 10% increased probability for them to do so within the first week after the primary cardiovascular event. Several different measures can help to decrease this risk or reduce the severity of the recurrent stroke; one of which is the use of aspirin.

For a long time now, physicians and scientists have recommended taking aspirin immediately after minor or major strokes. It has been shown that even a daily dose of 30 mg/day can aid those at risk of recurrent strokes.

Males and females of all ages can benefit from this strategy, since it is age and sex-independent. The importance of taking aspirin right after a stroke has been highly remarked. Minor strokes can have subtle symptoms and the patient can suffer from a secondary stroke while looking for medical attention, therefore, even when a stroke is only suspected, aspirin treatment is recommended.

Tip #1

▶ Immediately initiating a treatment of at least 30 mg of aspirin per day after a possible stroke

▶ Even minor strokes can have severe consequences - emergency services should be contacted immediately

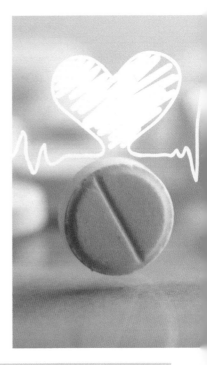

Organisations
My Stroke Guide - https://go22.uk/stroke1
The Stroke Association gives you free access to trusted information about different types of stroke, risk factors and secondary conditions, as well as advice on prevention and improving your own health.

Information
NHS Learn to Act F.A.S.T. - https://go22.uk/stroke2
Do you know the signs of a stroke? Knowing what to look out for could save someone's life, or even your own.

Effects of aspirin on risk and severity of early recurrent stroke after transient ischemic attack and ischemic stroke: time-course analysis of randomised trials
The Lancet - https://go22.uk/rp0011
The considerable early benefit from aspirin warrants public education about self-administration

COST: ● ● ● ● ○   EASE: ● ● ● ○ ○   IMPACT: ● ● ● ○ ○

Defibrillators

Many deaths occur following out-of-hospital cardiac arrests. The British Heart Foundation registers more than 30,000 out-of-hospital cardiac arrests in the UK each year and, unfortunately, the overall survival rate is less than one in ten.

However, the survival chances jump with a defibrillator. If a defibrillator is used within 3-5 minutes of the cardiac arrest, then the survival rate jumps to around six in ten.

Cardiac arrest results from an electrical disturbance in heart, which disrupts the pumping action and blood flow - the person becomes unconscious and unresponsive and cannot breathe normally.

If someone has had a cardiac arrest:
1. Call for an ambulance
2. Start CPR
3. Find out if there is a defibrillator nearby

With an automated external defibrillator (AED) anyone can help someone having a cardiac arrest.
- Attach the two electrode pads of the defibrillator to the patient's bare chest.
- The device will analyse the heart's electrical rhythm and deliver a shock.
- Modern defibrillators provide audible and even visual instructions regarding CPR.
Keep in mind that defibrillation is crucial in the chain of survival and that modern defibrillators will not allow a shock to be given unless needed.

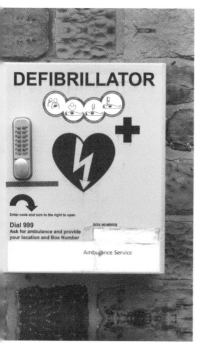

▷ **Campaign for defibrillators to be installed at your workplace and local public places**

▷ **Attend a CPR (cardiopulmonary resuscitation) training course**

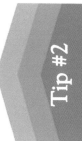

Tip #2

Information

About defibrillators - British Heart Foundation advice on defibrillators and cardiac arrest - https://go22.uk/bhfdef

How to Use a Defibrillator (AED) training video from St John Ambulance - https://go22.uk/sjadef

Products

Defibrillators - https://go22.uk/defibs
Defibshop has sold over 20,000 defibrillators to companies large or small, leisure centres and even households.

National initiatives to improve outcomes from out-of-hospital cardiac arrest in England
Emergency Medicine Journal - https://go22.uk/rp0491
Defibrillation within 3–5 min can produce survival rates as high as 50%–70%.
BHF CVD Statistics Compendium 2017
British Heart Foundation - https://go22.uk/rp0492
Including out-of-hospital cardiac arrest survival rates, England 2011-12 to 2015-16

COST: ● ● ● ○ ○   EASE: ● ● ● ○ ○   IMPACT: ● ● ○ ○ ○

Drowning prevention

Enjoy the refreshing water in summer, but pay attention because drowning is a leading cause of accidental death. In the UK, 265 people (excluding crime and suicide) drowned in 2016. The number is decreasing (from 321 in 2015), but the National Water Safety Forum states that caution is needed, as many of those who died did not even intend to be in the water: over a quarter of those deaths were walkers/runners and 5% were angling.

Be aware of bank edges, which are often unstable, and of incoming tides. If unfamiliar with the area go with a friend, who can help in case of difficulty.

Test the temperature of fresh water lakes and rivers; always enter feet first in order to prevent hypothermia and injuries due to rocks; never swim in a strong current. In the sea, pay attention to riptides.

If you are in danger of drowning, keeping calm is most important; first, move your legs in a scissor motion in order to reach the surface and control your breathing by inhaling when your head emerges from the water; float in order to save energy or gently tread water.

DON'T DRINK AND DROWN
Research by the Royal Life Saving Society found that 29% of all accidental drownings involved alcohol and/or drugs.

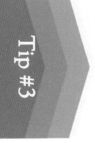

Tip #3

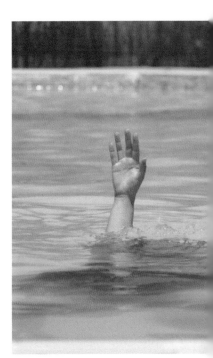

▶ Learn basic swimming skills: treading water, flotation and crawl stroke
▶ Buy only certified flotation devices and check them periodically
▶ Install underwater alarms in private and public pools

Information
Royal Yachting Association (RYA) advice including levels of buoyancy information sheet and how to wear a lifejacket correctly video - https://go22.uk/lifejackets

Products
Residential pools Drowning Detection Systems BlueFox – bracelet monitors the wearer's actual behaviour - https://go22.uk/bluefox
Coral Detection Systems - computer vision based - https://go22.uk/coraldds

WAID (WAter Incident Database) Reports - https://go22.uk/rp1061
The reports are compiled by members of the National Water Safety Forum and published on a calendar-year basis.

Drowning Prevention and Water Safety Week 2017
National Fire Chiefs Council - https://go22.uk/rp1062
For every drowning fatality there are 8 incidents which leave people with life changing injuries

COST: ● ● ● ○ ○ EASE: ● ● ● ● ● IMPACT: ● ● ● ● ●

Donate to longevity research

Even if you faithfully followed every tip in this book, at the moment that would only make you live longer (a good thing!) but not forever. Indefinite life extension relies on the first few generations of anti-ageing therapies arriving in time for you to reach longevity escape velocity.

However, because most government funding is focussed on specific diseases (such as cancer which, if cured, would only add a few years to life expectancy) the university teams researching the fundamental causes of ageing are generally underfunded.

It is critically important to fund this basic research as it has two main benefits. Firstly, the results are made freely available to other teams working on a wider range of subjects. For example, the MouseAge campaign by lifespan.io raised funds to create an AI-powered tool to determine the biological age of mice accurately, based on photographic images. This will help speed up the pace of longevity research in hundreds of laboratories around the world that use mice as their ageing model.

Secondly, it progresses the science to the point where companies get interested. Investors need to see returns within a shorter time frame, so won't risk their money until at least the basic mechanism has been proven. For example, Ichor Therapeutics is soon to run clinical trials of an enzyme that helps lysosomes in retinal pigment epithelium cells fight age-related macular degeneration – but that treatment relies on prior work by the SENS Research Foundation that proved the basic principles.

▷ Donate to Lifespan.io crowdfunding
  campaigns
▷ Donate to SENS Research Foundation

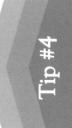

Tip #4

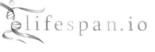

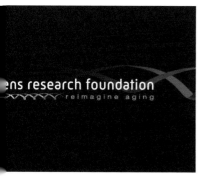

Organisations
Lifespan.io from the Life Extension Advocacy Foundation (LEAF)
https://go22.uk/leaf
Crowdfunding relevant research and advocating for its benefits to society.

SENS Research Foundation
https://go22.uk/sens
SENS Research Foundation is a 501(c)(3) public charity. Donations from residents of the USA are fully deductible as a charitable contribution.

MouseAge: Visual Biomarker for Mouse Aging
Lifespan.io - https://go22.uk/mouseage
Using AI and Computer Vision Techniques to Determine Age and Assess the Effect of Therapies

OncoSENS Control ALT Delete Cancer
Lifespan.io - https://go22.uk/altdelete
High-throughput screening of a library of diverse drugs to find treatments for 'ALT' cancers

COST: ● ● ● ● ●   EASE: ● ● ● ● ○   IMPACT: ● ● ● ● ○

Raise awareness of life extension

Along with the lack of funding, one of the biggest impediments to anti-ageing research is lack of interest or, often, complete resistance to the concept. Two common initial responses to the idea of living forever are, firstly, that it's impossible so why waste time discussing it, and secondly, the consequences would be so awful that it should not even be contemplated. Both arguments attempt to invalidate any further debate, however, until people start discussing the subject, these reflex responses won't change.

It may be that people are so culturally accustomed to death, and understandably so as up to this point in time it has been an absolute certainty, that it is just too difficult a change of direction. But even a supertanker changes direction when given enough time. So it's important that the subject is raised as often as possible, to highlight that scientific advances, which don't make the headlines, are slowly chipping away at the causes of ageing, and that it could well be possible to live long enough to be here when it is cured.

The magnitude of the coming longevity revolution does make it hard to convince people of its validity, though equally, once persuaded, this makes it a topic people are keen to share with others. So as more people see the light, pressure will build on governments to provide more funding for research and the demand will tempt more investors to set up companies to provide new treatments.

Tip #5

▶ Bring the subject up in conversation – it always gets a lively response

▶ Share interesting developments on social media

▶ Join or follow the Live Forever Club to keep up with the latest news

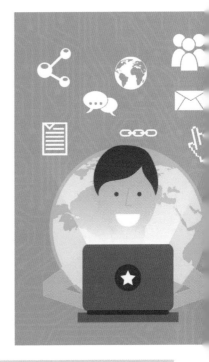

Organisations
Live Forever Club - https://go22.uk/club
Curates life extension news and useful resources with the aim of promoting equality in longevity

Meet up with like minded people to help develop your knowledge and arguments - https://go22.uk/meetup

Information
Frequently Asked Questions on the Ethics of Lifespan and Healthspan Extension by Ilia Stambler for the Institute for Ethics and Emerging Technologies - https://go22.uk/ieetfaq

The Fable of the Dragon-Tyrant
YouTube - https://go22.uk/fable
Animated version of Nick Bostrom's philosophical parable about death. How a planet ravaged by a dragon demands the sacrifice of thousands of people every day and how most people accepted the inevitable.

COST: ● ● ● ● ●   EASE: ● ● ● ○ ○   IMPACT: ● ● ● ● ○

Alcohol

There's a great deal of controversy regarding alcohol. Numerous epidemiological studies have found a protective effect of moderate alcohol consumption, while there is considerable evidence pointing against it. Where studies found not drinking at all was less healthy than moderate consumption this may be have been because of sick quitters' bias – teetotallers included former alcoholics and people already too sick to drink.

Some scientists have showed that small amounts of alcohol in your diet may lower the risk of some cardiovascular outcomes, such as stroke, coronary heart disease etc. On the other hand, emerging data links different types of cancer with alcohol (including mouth, throat and breast). It is possible that alcohol isn't itself a carcinogen but that it promotes the effects of other carcinogens, at least in the digestive tract.

Furthermore, women might be more vulnerable during their pre/postmenopausal period - a study involving 556 postmenopausal women concluded that those who started drinking before the age of 40 had a 2.5 higher risk of breast cancer occurrence than never-drinkers.

A 30 year-long Harvard University study has also shown a six-fold increase in the risk of hippocampal brain shrinkage, which can affect long-term memory, for those having four or more drinks a day.

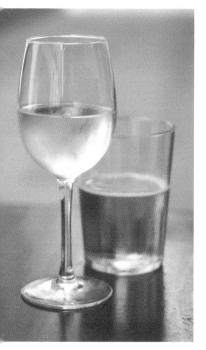

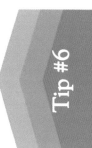

▷ Consider the guidance levels as a maximum and aim to drink less
▷ Have several drink-free days each week

Tip #6

Information

UK Chief Medical Officers' guidelines
https://go22.uk/alcohol1

Alcohol units - quick guide to work out how many units are in your favourite tipple
NHS - https://go22.uk/alcohol2

UK Chief Medical Officers' Low Risk Drinking Guidelines
Department of Health - https://go22.uk/rp0341
Detailed background to guidelines and the evidence considered by the expert group

Alcohol use and burden for 195 countries and territories, 1990–2016: a systematic analysis for the Global Burden of Disease Study 2016
The Lancet - https://go22.uk/rp0342

COST: ●●●○○   EASE: ●●●●●   IMPACT: ●●○○○

Aluminium cookware

Aluminium is present in soil, rocks, and clay. But did you know that you consume extra amounts of aluminium without being aware of it? You ingest it when drinking from cans or when you eat a dish prepared in aluminium cookware.

Many studies have confirmed that this metal can leach out from pots and pans. But it depends on what you cook and how long for. Your meals will contain more aluminium if you cook something acidic, such as tomato sauce, compared to when you cook low acid foods such as meat.

Be aware of aluminium foil - use it for food storage only. Dishes prepared in it may absorb even more of the metal. Study groups found that a small amount of aluminium leaches from drink cans after some time too.

Science doesn't say much about the impact of aluminium leaching from cookware, but there are many studies that have investigated the health effects of tap water aluminium. Too much of it may affect the central nervous system in a bad way and populations that consume drinking water high in aluminium are more likely to develop dementia.

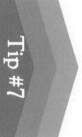

Tip #7

▶ Use alternative cookware (e.g. stainless steel, glass, enamel) for very acid foods
▶ Avoid storing food in aluminium containers or foil
▶ Replace damaged aluminium pans

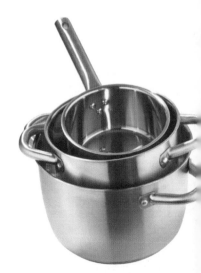

Information
Benefits and risks of cookware materials
https://go22.uk/cookware
Canadian government highlights potential risks in some cookware materials, and how to minimise them.

European Food Safety Authority - https://go22.uk/rp1141
Safety of aluminium from dietary intake - Scientific Opinion of the Panel on Food Additives, Flavourings, Processing Aids and Food Contact Materials (AFC)

Relation between aluminum concentrations in drinking water and Alzheimer's disease
American Journal of Epidemiology - https://go22.uk/rp1142
High levels (>0.1 mg/l) were associated with an elevated risk of dementia and Alzheimer's

COST: ● ● ● ● ●   EASE: ● ● ● ● ○   IMPACT: ● ● ● ○ ○

Artificial sweeteners

Artificial sweeteners are sugar replacers commonly found in drinks and food products. The most consumed ones in the UK are acesulfame K, aspartame, saccharin, sorbitol, sucralose, stevia and xylitol.

There has been considerable debate about their potential carcinogenic impact, however, EFSA and other regulatory bodies have discarded this view as there is insufficient evidence to support.

Although it has been established that they are safe for consumption, there is evidence that they might promote weight gain. In fact, artificial sweeteners can change the way the body responds (such as hormones that regulate our food intake) when eating something sweet. These changes may eventually cause the body to respond differently when consuming real sugar which can lead to overeating and weight gain.

A recent meta-analysis established that heavy consumers of artificial sweeteners are at greater risk of diabetes type 2, metabolic syndrome and elevated blood pressure. A different study found that a high intake of artificially sweetened products is a significant contributor in triggering dementia and stroke.

So, although they're not carcinogenic, it is still better to avoid artificial sweeteners where possible.

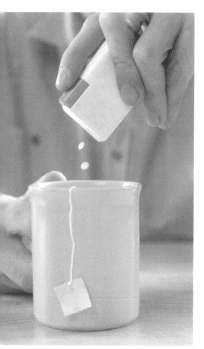

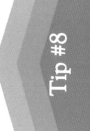

Tip #8

▷ Keep consumption of artificially sweetened drinks to less than 5 a week
▷ Learn to love tea and coffee without artificial sweeteners
▷ Watch what you're eating/drinking – check the label for hidden sweeteners

Information

Artificial Sweeteners and Cancer - https://go22.uk/sweeteners1
Fact sheet from the National Cancer Institute including what studies have shown about specific artificial sweeteners.

High-Intensity Sweeteners Permitted for Use in Food in the United States - https://go22.uk/sweeteners2
FDA summary table includes brand names, their multiplier of sweetness intensity and Acceptable Daily Intake (ADI).

Nonnutritive sweeteners and cardiometabolic health: a systematic review and meta-analysis CMAJ - https://go22.uk/rp0921
Consumption of nonnutritive sweeteners is associated with higher risks of obesity, hypertension, metabolic syndrome, type 2 diabetes, stroke and cardiovascular disease events.

Sugar- and Artificially Sweetened Beverages and the Risks of Incident Stroke and Dementia Stroke - https://go22.uk/rp0922

COST: ●●● ○ ○   EASE: ●● ○ ○ ○   IMPACT: ●●●● ○

Calorie restriction

Many animal studies confirm that calorie restriction might slow ageing by lowering the concentrations of biomarkers linked to ageing-associated diseases. In human studies, however, these kinds of results should always be interpreted cautiously, as they are less precise because they cannot monitor human subjects in an isolated environment.

Calorie restriction is not simply eating a little less, it is a dramatic reduction of calorie intake to the point where it requires significant planning to meet the body's nutritional needs - undernutrition without malnutrition.

Epidemiological data reports that men and women in Okinawa, Japan, possess among the highest functional capacities and the longest survival in the country, which has world's longest-living population. This data points out that their low calorie intake (15% less than Japan's average) might be the explanation for long life expectancy and the high prevalence of centenarians.

However, not all data supports this theory, as some animal studies found that subjects following a calorie restriction programme ended with a compromised immune system and infertility. This has not yet been observed in human trials.

So far, it has been confirmed that long-term reduced calorie intake lowers insulin and cholesterol levels, and improves general and mental health in subjects who have undergone months or years of calorie restriction (but not severe restriction which can have adverse effects).

Tip #9

▶ Aim for a body fat percentage of 10/18% (male/female)

▶ Eat foods that are high in nutrients but low in calories

▶ Join the CR Society International for support and advice

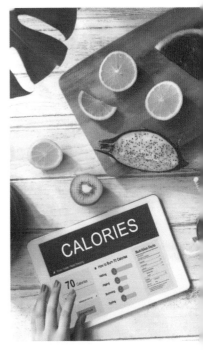

Organisations
CR Society - https://go22.uk/crsociety
Formed in 1994 the CR Society supports the efforts of people who practice calorie restriction.
Includes forums, scientific research and in-depth resources.

Effect of CR on Mood, Quality of Life, Sleep, and Sexual Function in Healthy Nonobese Adults
JAMA Internal Medicine - https://go22.uk/rp0151
Analyses supported the association between weight loss & improved health-related quality of life

Long-term calorie restriction is highly effective in reducing the risk for atherosclerosis in humans
Proceedings of the National Academy of Sciences - https://go22.uk/rp0152
Sustained beneficial effects on cholesterol, triglycerides and blood pressure

COST: ● ● ● ● ●   EASE: ● ● ● ● ○   IMPACT: ● ● ● ○ ○

Chilli peppers (capsaicin)

Chilli peppers serve as an abundant source of minerals, vitamins and antioxidants which makes them an ideal ingredient in a healthy diet.

One of the main compounds in chillies is capsaicin. It is this alkaloid compound which is responsible for the pungent and spicy character of chilli. However, chilli also owes its health benefits to capsaicin, as a number of laboratory studies have shown that it possesses anti-bacterial, anti-carcinogenic, anti-diabetic and analgesic properties. This wonder compound enhances the metabolic rate, diminishes appetite and boosts fat oxidation, making chillies an ideal component of a balanced weight loss diet. It has also been shown to reduce bad cholesterol in the body thereby, paving the way to better cardiovascular health.

Consumption of chillies has been associated with longer life. Two independent studies showed that the mortality rate of people who consumed chillies, at least once or twice a week, was 10-12% lower than the people who ate spicy food less often. It was even lower for people who consumed spicy food almost every day.

A common myth is that chillies cause gastric ulcers. On the contrary, if consumed in moderate amounts they not only prevent but also aid healing of gastric ulcers. However, excessive consumption of chillies does lead to stomach discomfort.

Various other health benefits associated with chillies are reduction in inflammation and pain, clearing congestion and preventing spread of prostate cancer.

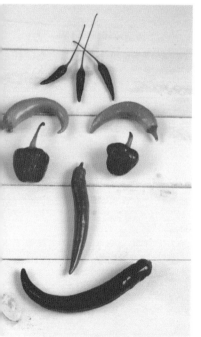

▷ Include a moderate amount of chilli peppers in your diet every day
▷ Try with a small amount of yogurt if you are not used to eating it

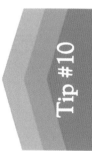

Tip #10

Information

Is the chilli pepper friend or foe? BBC Health Check
https://go22.uk/chilli

How Hot is That Pepper? How Scientists Measure Spiciness - Smithsonian magazine
https://go22.uk/scoville
Tabasco sauce has 5,000 Scoville heat units or SHU

Why Are Hot Peppers Hot? (And How Milk Helps) - American Chemical Society
https://go22.uk/capsaicin
Video explaining what capsaicin is and how it works

The Association of Hot Red Chili Pepper Consumption and Mortality
PLOS ONE - https://go22.uk/rp0161
Consumption of hot red chilli pepper increases life expectancy

Capsaicin may have important potential for promoting vascular and metabolic health
Open Heart - https://go22.uk/rp0162
Such as better cardiovascular health, weight loss and increased metabolic rate

COST: ●●●● ○   EASE: ●●●●●   IMPACT: ●● ○○○

Chocolate

Chocolate may not generally be considered a healthy food, particularly because of the high amount of added sugars, however, it also contains quite a few beneficial compounds if you pick the right type of chocolate.

Cocoa and cocoa-related products have an abundance of very powerful antioxidants - flavanols, which act like scavengers, catching the deleterious free radicals that cause harm to our inner cells and tissues and might promote many adverse health conditions.

Epidemiological studies provide strong evidence for flavanols' positive effect on the cardiovascular system, and that consumption could lower LDL-cholesterol, blood pressure, the activity of platelets and improve endothelial function. In addition, heart attack patients who consumed chocolate a few times per week were shown to be at a lower risk of dying from cardiac disease compared with those who did not.

Eating a piece of chocolate may improve concentration - bioactive flavanols can increase blood flow in response to a cognitive task and this is seen in both elderly and young participants. These polyphenols are also involved in the protection and regeneration of neurons in the brain.

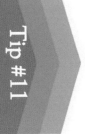

Tip #11

▶ Opt for dark chocolate with more than 70% of cocoa
▶ The best time for chocolate is after lunch when enzymes break sugar more efficiently

Products

Acticoa chocolate - https://go22.uk/acticoa
The only chocolate with an EU approved health claim. Acticoa's processing retains five times the cocoa flavanols of normal processes.

CocoaVia from Mars - https://go22.uk/cocoavia
Guarantees the highest concentration of cocoa flavanols available in a supplement.

Information

Dark Chocolate and Health - The Nutrition Source (Harvard University) - https://go22.uk/chocolate

Effects of chocolate, cocoa, and flavan-3-ols on cardiovascular health
The American Journal of Clinical Nutrition - https://go22.uk/rp0641
Meta-analysis confirmed the beneficial effects on various cardiovascular parameters

Influence of habitual chocolate consumption over the Mini-Mental State Examination
Nutricion Hospitalaria - https://go22.uk/rp0642
Dark chocolate consumption might improve cognitive function among the older population

COST: ● ● ● ● ●　　　EASE: ● ● ● ● ○　　　IMPACT: ● ● ● ○ ○

Coffee and caffeine

Caffeine is a natural stimulant commonly found in coffee, tea and other beverages. It is mostly recognised for its boosting effect on the central nervous system, however there are many other benefits.

Many scientific studies reveal that regular caffeine consumption can decrease the risks of type 2 diabetes, cirrhosis, cardiovascular diseases and some types of cancer. Besides those, it can lower the incidence of Alzheimer's disease and depression. It is also reported that caffeine can influence our energy balance and metabolism and in that way speed weight loss.

After analysing several trials which included more than a million participants, scientists found that light coffee consumption (1-3 cups/day) could reduce the risk of all-cause mortality by 11%, while moderate drinking (3-5 cups/day) reduced it by 13%.

However, you should be aware of the short-term adverse effects of caffeine such as increased blood pressure, interrupted sleep, anxiety and behavioural changes. In addition, pregnant women (because of their slower caffeine metabolism) must pay attention to their dietary habits, because data consistently confirms that excess caffeine consumption is related to low birth weight, pregnancy loss and childhood leukaemia.

Strangely, decaffeinated coffee consumption is also found to be associated with a lower risk of death, but the data is limited for these studies.

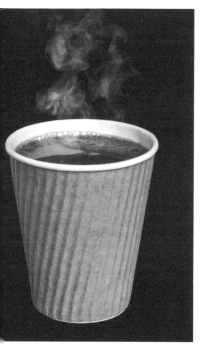

▷ Consume up to four cups of coffee day
▷ Drink high-caffeine beverages after a meal to avoid an unfavourable blood sugar response

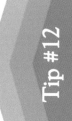

Tip #12

Information
Caffeine content for coffee, tea, soda and more
https://go22.uk/caffeine
Mayo Clinic chart highlights:
1. There is 2-5 times as much caffeine in a cup of coffee than in a cup of tea.
2. A can of Coke has about the same amount of caffeine as a cup of tea.

Association of coffee drinking with all-cause mortality: a systematic review and meta-analysis
Public Health Nutrition - https://go22.uk/rp0131
Light to moderate coffee consumption is associated with a reduced risk of death from all causes

Coffee, tea, caffeine and risk of depression: A systematic review
Molecular Nutrition & Food Research - https://go22.uk/rp0132
Coffee and caffeine consumption may exert a protective effect on the risk of depression.

COST: ● ● ● ● ●　　　EASE: ● ● ● ● ●　　　IMPACT: ● ● ○ ○ ○

Drink temperature

The International Agency for Research on Cancer raised a public concern in 2016, regarding the consumption of very hot beverages (coffee, tea, mate) and cancer. The evidence came from countries with an increasing prevalence of oesophageal cancer, which is estimated to cause around 5% of all cancer deaths.

Most of the large-scale studies investigating the link between oesophageal cancer and hot drink consumption were carried out in China, Turkey, and South America, which are all countries where beverages are regularly consumed at temperatures around 70°C. The World Health Organisation (WHO) warns that drinks above 65°C (149°F) are in the danger zone.

A possible way that hot drinks injure our body is by substantially increasing the temperature of the oesophageal inner layer, that way inducing stress and damaging the layer structure and function.

It is not yet clear quite how big the risk is, but, as an example, a study done in Iran reported that people who drank tea two or three minutes after it was poured compared with people who waited for five minutes or more had a 2.5 greater risk of oesophageal cancer, while those who drank it after less than two minutes had a 5.4 higher risk.

Tip #13

▶ Let your coffee/tea cool to below 65 °C (150 °F) before drinking it

▶ Milk or cold water should drop the temperature by 5-10 °C (10-20 °F)

▶ Use a smart mug/kettle to get the temperature right

Products

Bosch Styline Kettle – £69.99 (~US$91.59) - https://go22.uk/styline
Choose from four temperature settings at the correct temperatures.

Ember Temperature Control Mug - £79.95 (US$79.95) - https://go22.uk/embermug
Set your drink temperature between 50 °C - 62.5 °C.

Glowstone Mug - £129 (~US$168) - https://go22.uk/glowstone
Maintains drink temperature between 60° C to 65°C for an extra hour.

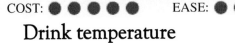

Is temperature an effect modifier of the association between green tea intake and gastric cancer risk? - European Journal of Cancer Prevention - https://go22.uk/rp0141
Hot tea consumption was linked with an increased risk of this disease.

Tea drinking habits and oesophageal cancer in a high-risk area in northern Iran BMJ - https://go22.uk/rp0142
Drinking hot tea was strongly associated with a higher risk of oesophageal cancer.

COST: ● ● ● ● ○   EASE: ● ● ● ● ○   IMPACT: ● ● ○ ○ ○

Fermented vegetables

Centuries ago our ancestors had to find a way to preserve vegetables. However, they weren't aware of the nutritional value of the dish they were making. Nowadays, the scientific and manufacturing community praise these food products for many reasons.

Firstly, fermented vegetables have a different, improved structure and digestibility. Secondly, they are abundant in vitamins, minerals, fibres, enzymes, and natural probiotics. These compounds can exert various health-promoting effects. They can help boost the immunity, lower cholesterol, atherosclerosis, inflammation and maintain weight.

Fermentation is not the same as pickling, which generally refers to preserving in vinegar. Fermented food creates its own acidic medium through lactic acid fermentation.

Epidemiological studies showed that people who ate sauerkraut at least once a week had a 20% lower risk of cancer. By eating fermented vegetables every day, we could lower the prevalence of stroke mortality by 35%.

However, fermented vegetables might have higher levels of salt (depending on the production process) and too much salt can cause detrimental health effects, so be careful to read the label.

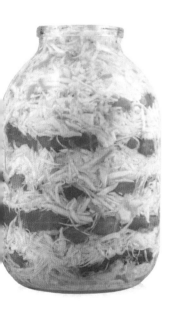

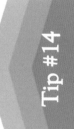

▶ Add some fermented vegetables, for example sauerkraut, to your daily diet
▶ Don't be put off the first time you try it! It can be an acquired taste which people come to like

Tip #14

Information
Fermenting Food UK - https://go22.uk/fermenting
Blog, guides and videos on how to do it yourself.

Products
Hengstenberg Bavarian Style Sauerkraut - £2.40/kg (US$3.10/kg) - https://go22.uk/fermented1
Germany's most popular sauerkraut and great value

No.1 Kombucha - £1.95 (US$2.50) - https://go22.uk/fermented2
Fermented green tea, bacteria and yeast, blended with fruit juice and botanicals for flavour.

The relationship between fermented food intake and mortality risk
British Journal of Nutrition - https://go22.uk/rp0931
Fermented vegetable intake was associated with a reduced risk of all-cause mortality.

Prospective study of fruit and vegetable intake and risk of prostate cancer
JNCI: Journal of the National Cancer Institute - https://go22.uk/rp0932
Higher sauerkraut and cabbage intake was associated with a lower risk of extraprostatic cancer.

COST: ●●●●●   EASE: ●●●●○   IMPACT: ●●○○○

Food hygiene

3,000 people die every year in the US (500 in the UK) from foodborne illness. Microorganisms are everywhere – they are present on and in our bodies, foods, drinks, etc. They include desirable, good species, whereas some of them are very bad, such as Salmonella, E.Coli and noroviruses.

The main cause of foodborne illnesses is bad hygiene (both food and personal) and the consequences are almost always very unpleasant. The symptoms involve vomiting, diarrhoea, stomach sickness and cramps, which finally make you dehydrated. The consequences are usually not fatal, however, there are reported cases of deaths due to food contamination, while the number of hospitalised people is not negligible.

In 2015, 18% of reported food hygiene incidents were caused by food pathogenic microorganisms, and 67% of them were due to the presence of Salmonella and E.Coli. A US study reported that the major contaminants that caused illness were plant-based products, while the largest percentage of deaths was provoked by land animal commodities (e.g. chicken) consumption. The statistics are somewhat different in the UK - a large survey found that people who ate poultry were admitted to hospitals more frequently, because of food poisoning, while fruits and vegetables had a minor or no impact on the occurrence of foodborne diseases.

Tip #15

▶ Keep raw meat away from ready-to-eat food (e.g. separate chopping boards)
▶ Cook food until it has reached 70 °C (160 °F) for at least two minutes
▶ Wash your hands before preparing food

Information
20 Ways You Can Get Food Poisoning
WebMD slideshow - https://go22.uk/food1

Organisations
Food Standards Agency - https://go22.uk/fsaUK
government department that protects public health
and consumers' wider interests in food.
Site includes guides, news and food recall alerts.

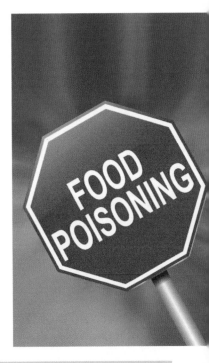

Disease Risks from Foods, England and Wales, 1996–2000
Emerging Infectious Diseases - https://go22.uk/rp0711
When all parameters were considered, infection due to chicken was consistently responsible for more disease, while disease linked to plant-based foods had a minor impact on the population.

COST: ● ● ● ○ ○   EASE: ● ● ● ● ○   IMPACT: ● ● ● ● ○

Fruit and vegetables

Fruits and vegetables are well-known sources of nutrients and their higher intake can prevent numerous adverse health conditions. The scientific evidence, that has been gathered from millions of people, in thousands of studies, conclusively shows that the consumption of fruits and vegetables increases life expectancy, and generally that the more that is eaten the greater the effect. Governments and the World Health Organisation guidelines recommend 400 grams per day (also known as "five-a-day"), although a 2017 summary analysis of large studies points out that eating twice as much could have an even better effect on longevity.

Epidemiological studies, looking at the associations between high fruit and vegetable consumption and specific risks/mortalities, find that they can reduce the risk of a wide range of diseases including cardiovascular disease and cancer, which are the two most common causes of premature death worldwide. All these positive effects are mostly caused by the presence of different phytochemicals that act as antioxidants and capture the free radical molecules that can damage the body's cells.

The preparation method is also an important factor in the health benefits of fruit and vegetables - some studies find that people who eat more raw vegetables might have an even longer survival rate.

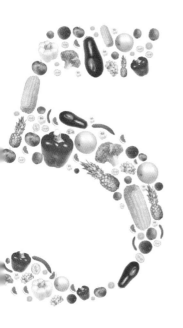

▷ Eat at least five portions of fruit & vegetables every day

▷ Have a mix of cooked and raw vegetables

▷ Wash all fruit and vegetables before you eat them

Tip #16

Information

How much is one serving?
American Heart Association - https://go22.uk/vegserving

Seasonality table
BBC Good Food - https://go22.uk/seasonality
See what's in season year-round

How to wash fruit and vegetables
NHS - https://go22.uk/washfruit
Advice on storing, washing and preparing fruit and vegetables to prevent food poisoning

Fruit and vegetable consumption and all-cause, cancer and CVD mortality
Journal of Epidemiology and Community Health - https://go22.uk/rp0371
Eating 7+ portions of fruit and vegetables daily have the lowest risk of mortality from any cause

Fruit and vegetable intake and cause-specific mortality in the EPIC study
European Journal of Epidemiology - https://go22.uk/rp0372
Associations were more pronounced for consumption of raw vegetables

COST: ● ● ● ● ●   EASE: ● ● ● ○ ○   IMPACT: ● ● ○ ○ ○

Garlic

Garlic has a long history as a mighty remedy that can boost immunity, treat infections, protect gastrointestinal health, and more. The first documented cases of garlic application come from Chinese traditional medicine, where it was recommended for curing poisoning.

Results of randomised controlled trials that have investigated the effects of garlic supplements found that they can lower blood pressure in people with or without hypertension and this in turn improves our cardiovascular health. While the results regarding garlic and lipid profile (cholesterol and triglycerides in the blood) are not consistent, evidence does show that people are at lower risk of developing colorectal cancers, if they consume garlic at least two times per week.

The secret beneath garlic's superpower might be in one part due to allicin - the main component responsible for its distinct smell. Other fighters in garlic's powerful army are manganese, vitamin B6 and vitamin C.

Garlic's health-promoting properties have been confirmed in many scientific studies where researchers have found that garlic supplements may enhance athletic performance and also reduce the chances of developing Alzheimer's disease and dementia.

Tip #17

▶ Make garlic a standard ingredient in most of your recipes.

▶ If your diet is lacking in garlic use supplements instead

▶ Combat the common cold with raw garlic combined with lemon and ginger

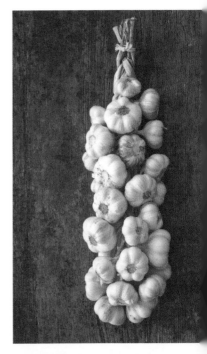

Information
Garlic drug interaction warnings
WebMD - https://go22.uk/garlic1
Including Isoniazid (Nydrazid, INH), Saquinavir (Fortovase, Invirase) and medications used for HIV/AIDS.

The Health Benefits of GarlicConsumer Reports - https://go22.uk/garlic2Including How to Get the Most Out of Garlic:
- Choose the freshest bulbs
- Store it right
- Chop it for your health

Garlic consumption and cancer prevention: meta-analyses of colorectal and stomach cancers. American Journal of Clinical Nutrition - https://go22.uk/rp0671
The published epidemiologic evidence suggests that protection against stomach and colorectal cancers is conferred by consumption of raw and cooked garlic.

Garlic Lowers Blood Pressure in Hypertensive Individuals, Regulates Serum Cholesterol, and Stimulates Immunity - The Journal of Nutrition - https://go22.uk/rp0672

COST: ● ● ● ● ●   EASE: ● ● ● ● ●   IMPACT: ● ● ○ ○ ○

Low temperature cooking

Scientific papers warn that roasted and fried starchy food contains a compound that may pose a risk to our health. This potential carcinogenic, acrylamide, is a product created by the reaction between amino acids and sugars at temperatures higher than 120 °C (250 °F).

Acrylamide can be found in many foods including potatoes, breakfast cereals, chips, biscuits, coffee, black olives, and root vegetables. The results of animal studies revealed that acrylamide may increase the risk of various types of cancer, but prospective human studies report inconsistent results.

The International Agency for Research on Cancer (IARC) classifies acrylamide as a "probable human carcinogen" based on the animal studies' data, while it confirms that data from human trials are "inadequate" to draw a conclusion. However, epidemiological data supports the link between high acrylamide intake and increased risk of endometrial and ovarian cancer in women.

The UK government's Food Standard Agency has developed guidelines for commercial food manufacturers, to mitigate acrylamide formation in the food they produce, but it's also important to take measures of your own so as to reduce dietary acrylamide.

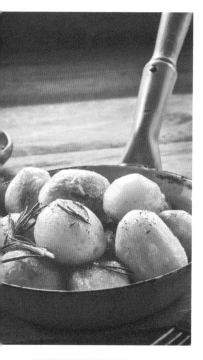

▷ Fried, roasted or baked starchy food should have a golden, not brown colour

▷ Follow the preparation instructions on purchased products

Tip #18

Information

What Food Products Contain Acrylamide?
Choices Magazine - https://go22.uk/acrylamide
Chart shows acrylamide content ranges from under 100 parts per billion (ppb) in vegetables and dairy products to over 1,000 ppb in snacks and chips.

Acrylamide in the home: the effects of home-cooking on acrylamide generation
Food Standard Agency research project - https://go22.uk/fsa2

A Prospective Study on Dietary Acrylamide Intake and the Risk for Breast, Endometrial, and Ovarian Cancers
Cancer Epidemiology, Biomarkers & Prevention - https://go22.uk/rp1081
Risk for endometrial cancer and possibly ovarian cancer was greater among high acrylamide consumers

COST: ● ● ● ● ●   EASE: ● ● ● ● ●   IMPACT: ● ● ● ○ ○

Milk

Milk has long been considered to be essential for bone health, although when it comes to hip fractures, studies don't support the view that drinking milk can lower their incidence; some report even higher fracture incidence and mortality rate in heavy milk drinkers.

Experimental data also warns that D-galactose (a milk sugar similar to lactose) may be detrimental to health. It has been found that chronic exposure to this sugar may cause inflammation, compromise the immune response and shorten lifespan. There is plenty of evidence that men are more likely to have prostate cancer if they consume high amounts of milk (three glasses per day or more), and have an increased mortality risk from cardiovascular and cancer.

However, there are also papers supporting that drinking some milk may be health promoting. One big-scale Japanese study suggests that people who consumed milk at least 3-4 times/week enhanced their survival rate compared with non-consumers, however, these benefits weren't seen to increase with more frequent consumption.

So the evidence, at present, suggests it is important to get the balance just right – regular, low-level consumption of milk to obtain its valuable nutrients but without overdoing it.

Tip #19

▶ Limit yourself to 1 glass of milk per day
▶ Use Greek yoghurt on cereals instead of milk
▶ Try dairy alternatives such as soya, almond or rice milk

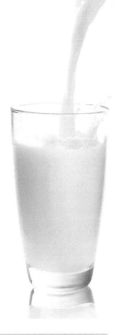

Information

Is Milk Good for Our Bones?
NutritionFacts.org - https://go22.uk/milkbones
Video explaining the current research into milk, bone fractures and life expectancy

Which milk is right for you? Review of dairy and non-dairy milk alternatives
BBC Good Food - https://go22.uk/whichmilk

Worldwide Total Milk Consumption per capita
ChartsBin - https://go22.uk/milkconsumption

Drinks to Consume in Moderation
Harvard University - https://go22.uk/moderation

Milk intake and risk of mortality and fractures in women and men: cohort studies
BMJ - https://go22.uk/rp1171
High milk intake was associated with higher mortality in women and men

Milk Drinking and Mortality: Findings From the Japan Collaborative Cohort Study
Journal of Epidemiology - https://go22.uk/rp1172
Drinking milk at least 1–2 times a month was associated with lower all-cause mortality

COST: ● ● ● ● ◦   EASE: ● ● ● ● ◦   IMPACT: ● ● ◦ ◦ ◦

Nuts

A large body of evidence suggests that nuts should definitely be included in our everyday diet. This particularly refers to almonds, walnuts, pistachios and hazelnuts. These have many powerful antioxidant, anti-inflammatory and antithrombotic properties.

Nuts are abundant in many health-promoting bioactive compounds such as mono- and polyunsaturated fatty acids, soluble fibre, vitamins (e.g. folate and vitamin E), minerals (e.g. magnesium and potassium), and phytochemicals (e.g. flavonoids and phytosterols).

Many epidemiological trials confirmed that eating nuts may be cardioprotective by imposing a positive effect on blood lipids, weight, and insulin resistance. It may lower the risk of diabetes, total and specific types of cancer, and can improve respiratory and neurological systems. All these features make nuts efficient longevity promoters.

They are a very important part of the famous Mediterranean diet; a group of scientists confirmed this by establishing a relationship between nuts and seeds intake and leukocyte telomere length, a biomarker of biological ageing.

Although high in fat, nuts contain healthy monounsaturated and polyunsaturated fats, and some also contain omega-3 fatty acids.

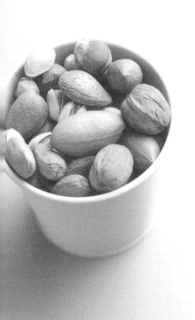

▶ Include 30 grams (1 ounce) of nuts in your daily diet

▶ Eat a variety of nuts such as almonds, walnuts and brazil nuts

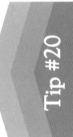

Tip #20

Information

Eating nuts for heart health
Mayo Clinic - https://go22.uk/nuts4heart
Includes a table of calorie and fat content for a variety of nuts

Nut eaters may have a longer life expectancy
NHS looks at the science behind the headlines - https://go22.uk/nhsnuts
Eating 28g of nuts seven or more times per week was associated with a 20% reduced risk of death

Nut consumption in relation to all-cause and cause-specific mortality: a meta-analysis 18 prospective studies
Food & Function - https://go22.uk/rp0681
High nut consumption was associated with lower risk of all-cause mortality with the greatest reduction being CHD mortality

COST: ● ● ● ○ ○   EASE: ● ● ● ● ○   IMPACT: ● ● ● ● ○

Pescatarian diet

Vegetarian diets (which include plenty of fruits, vegetables, nuts, etc.) can protect cardiovascular health, help maintain weight and sugar levels, and in that way promote longevity. However, it is not the healthiest possible diet. A pescatarian diet, which omits animal meat but combines the additional fruit and vegetable intake with the known health benefits of fish, seems to be the key to the longest lifespan.

A study of over 70,000 people found that compared to non-vegetarians, the risk of dying over a six-year period was reduced by the following:
Vegetarians = 9%
Vegans = 15%
Pescatarians = 19%

Fish has high levels of omega 3 fats and vitamin D which affect a vast range of metabolic pathways and help nourish the body.

For people who want to follow a vegan diet for ethical reasons, then it may be possible to reproduce the benefits of a pescatarian diet with foods and dietary supplements that mimic the benefits of fish.

Tip #21

▶ Avoid animal products in your diet
▶ Consume fish several times a week

Organisations
The Pescetarian Society - https://go22.uk/pescsoc
Providing a community based around a healthy but happy, natural diet for the mass population

Information
Vegetarian diet: How to get the best nutrition
Mayo Clinic - https://go22.uk/vegetrition
The more restrictive your diet is, the more challenging it can be to get all the nutrients you need

What is a pescatarian diet?
BBC Good Food - https://go22.uk/bbcpesc

Vegetarian dietary patterns and mortality in Adventist Health Study 2
JAMA Internal Medicine - https://go22.uk/rp0321
Lower mortality in all pesco-vegetarian, vegan, and lacto-ovo–vegetarian diets

Vegetarianism and breast, colorectal and prostate cancer risk
Journal of Human Nutrition and Dietetics - https://go22.uk/rp0322
Pesco-vegetarian diets were associated with a lower risk of colorectal cancer

COST: ● ● ● ● ○   EASE: ● ● ● ● ○   IMPACT: ● ● ○ ○ ○

Prebiotics and probiotics

In practice, probiotics refer to food supplemented with "good" bacteria. These are have been associated to health benefits that range from improving digestion to preventing cancer. Some studies have even linked probiotics to life extension in mice.

There are a wide variety of probiotics currently on the market but these can only bring significant benefits if they become a regular part of your diet since several of their effects are not long-lasting.

The food product may vary (yogurt, kefir, fermented milk, etc.) but the active component is microorganisms. The most common and well-known for their beneficial effects are Lactobacillus, Bifidobacterium, Streptococcus thermophilus and Saccharomyces.

Prebiotic refers to substances in foods that are not digested but end up intact in the colon where they serve as fuel for healthy gut microbiota. Onions, garlic, bananas, nuts, wholegrains and berries are excellent sources of prebiotics.

Using prebiotics and probiotics together ensures that good bacteria are present, and able to grow, in the gut.

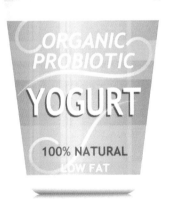

▶ Yogurt, apple cider vinegar and raw cheese are sources of good bacteria

▶ Supplement with probiotics and prebiotics if not present in your diet

▶ Consult your doctor first if you have predisposition for colitis

Tip #22

Information
The Microbiome and the role of probiotics
Harvard University - https://go22.uk/probiome

Products
Yakult - https://go22.uk/yakult
Fermented skimmed milk drink containing a strain of bacteria proven to reach the gut alive

Bimuno - https://go22.uk/bimuno
Galactooligosaccharide works by selectively increasing the level of bifidobacteria and other health-promoting bacteria found in the gut

Bifidobacterium longum, a lactic acid-producing intestinal bacterium inhibits colon cancer and modulates the intermediate biomarkers of colon carcinogenesis
Carcinogenesis - https://go22.uk/rp1021

Daily ingestion of fermented milk containing Lactobacillus casei DN114001 improves innate defense capacity in healthy middle-aged people
Journal of Physiology and Biochemistry - https://go22.uk/rp1022

COST: ●●●○○   EASE: ●●●○○   IMPACT: ●●●○○

Processed foods

The industrial era has brought with it a wide range of cheap, tempting products; however, it is important to be aware of their damaging effects. The main enemies in processed food are high amounts of added sugar and salt, as well as naturally present saturated fats.

Even worse than saturated fats are industrially-made trans fats. These increase levels of low-density lipoprotein ("bad" cholesterol) and promote inflammation, leading to increased risk of coronary heart disease, stroke, and diabetes, as well as a higher risk of overall mortality. Fortunately, consumer pressure and government regulations have reduced the amount of trans fat in food production, but not entirely, so it's important to always check the label.

Another harmful compound is furan, found in industrial heat-treated food products, a chemical contaminant that builds up in the liver, though further research is needed to determine a safe level.

In general, high consumption of processed meat (e.g. bacon, sausages, ham, salami, jerky) is associated with hypertension, heart disease and bowel cancer, and more than doubles the risk of colorectal cancer.

Tip #23

▶ Cook using fresh ingredients instead of processed foodstuffs

▶ Don't eat at a fast-food restaurant more than once a month

▶ Plan in advance to avoid resorting to convenience food

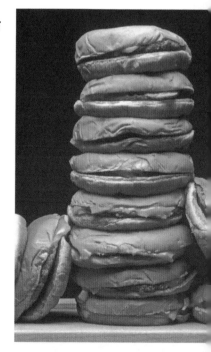

Information
6 Worst Trans Fat Foods You Commonly Consume
University Health News -
https://go22.uk/transfatfoods

Good fats and bad fats explained
British Nutrition Foundation -
https://go22.uk/badfats
Different types of fat, including the current fad for
coconut oil, and what they mean to your health

Intake of saturated and trans unsaturated fatty acids and risk of all cause mortality, cardiovascular disease, and type 2 diabetes
BMJ - https://go22.uk/rp0361

Risk of colorectal and other gastro-intestinal cancers after exposure to nitrate, nitrite and N-nitroso compounds
International Journal of Cancer - https://go22.uk/rp0362

COST: ●●●●●   EASE: ●●●●○   IMPACT: ●●●○○

Salt

High blood pressure is a major modifiable risk factor in cardiovascular disease, and clinical trials clearly show that excess salt and sodium consumption are significant contributors. There is also evidence that high salt intake may promote the progress of some other chronic diseases and types of cancer.

Reducing salt intake by one teaspoon (5 grams) per day has been shown to lower blood pressure by 4 mm Hg in people who are hypertensive (i.e. have high blood pressure). Unfortunately, the most recent report, from 2014, shows that the average salt consumption in adults in the UK was 8.0 g/day - 11% lower than the 2006 survey, but still 33% higher than the recommended 6g/day. It's estimated that a reduction in salt from 8 to 6 g/day could prevent 8000 premature deaths, annually.

When checking the salt content of foods, don't be tricked where manufacturers state sodium levels instead of salt – it's not the same thing. Sodium chloride is the chemical name for salt, hence sodium is just a part of it. To convert sodium to salt content, multiply the sodium amount by 2.5. For example, 1g of sodium per 100g is 2.5 grams of salt per 100g – that's a big difference.

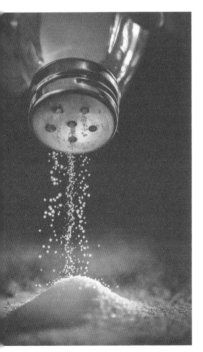

▷ Keep salt intake below the 6 grams daily allowance

▷ Substitute salt with other flavourful herbs and spices in your cooking

▷ Always check the label for salt content

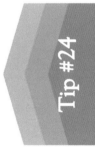

Tip #24

Information

Salt: the facts
NHS - https://go22.uk/nhssalt

Low-salt recipes
Blood Pressure UK - https://go22.uk/lowsalt

19 natural salt alternatives
British Heart Foundation - https://go22.uk/saltalter
With instructions on how to use them with meat, fish and vegetables

Salt intake, stroke, and cardiovascular disease: meta-analysis of prospective studies
BMJ - https://go22.uk/rp0171
People consuming high amounts of salt had 1.23 greater risk of having a stroke, and 1.14 times more chance of cardiovascular disease, than people consuming less salty food

COST: ● ● ● ● ●   EASE: ● ● ● ○ ○   IMPACT: ● ● ● ● ○

Sugar

When people talk about sugar they usually think about simple sugars - the good ones present in fruits and also the bad added sugar. Sugar is essential as it serves as a fuel for the body and provides energy; however, it should be consumed as fruit, not processed sweet products.

Scientific findings regarding added sugar are straightforward - eating it increases the risk of cardiovascular disease, metabolic syndrome, diabetes, and cancer, as well as the overall mortality risk. In addition, excessive sugar consumption acidifies the environment in the mouth and consequently makes it attractive for unfavourable bacteria which cause tooth decay.

Fructose is often added to processed foods in the form of corn syrup. High sugar diets, particularly those in high in fructose, also increase the risk of becoming leptin resistant. Leptin is the satiety hormone that tells the body when it has enough energy, so losing this signal means the brain is always hungry, encouraging people to eat more, creating a vicious circle. Thankfully the fibre in whole fruits slows down the release of sugar in the body so does not have the same effect.

Despite these facts, people in the UK tend to consume 2.5 times more than the recommended 5% of daily intake.

Tip #25

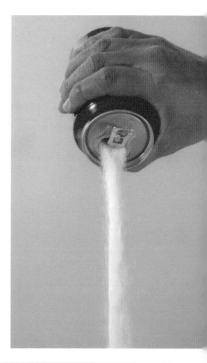

▶ Keep added sugar below 5% of your total diet (about 30 grams per day)

▶ Cut out fizzy drinks – some cans contain 9 teaspoons (45 g) of sugar

▶ Check the label - low fat products often add extra sugar to compensate

Information

How to cut down on sugar in your diet
NHS Eat Well guide - https://go22.uk/nhssugar

Infographic: how much sugar is in different foods?
British Heart Foundation -
https://go22.uk/howmuchsugar

Is Fructose Bad for You? Here's Why Fructose Is Worse Than Sugar
University Health News - https://go22.uk/fructose

Added Sugar Intake and Cardiovascular Diseases Mortality Among US Adults
JAMA Internal Medicine - https://go22.uk/rp0651
Risk was more than double for those consuming more than 20% of calories from added sugar

Sugar and artificially sweetened soda consumption linked to hypertension
Clinical and Experimental Hypertension - https://go22.uk/rp0652
Meta-analysis showed a significant association between soda consumption and hypertension

COST: ● ● ● ● ○   EASE: ● ● ● ● ○   IMPACT: ● ● ● ○ ○

Wholegrains

Large-scale studies report that people who consume higher amounts of wholegrains and their products are more likely to have a lower risk of adverse cardiovascular outcomes, different types of cancer and overall mortality.

Wholegrains are abundant in many nutritious components such as fibre, B vitamins and antioxidants which all nourish the body. There is a wide range of different grains: wheat, oats, maize, rye, and pseudocereals (buckwheat). Ancient grains (sorghum, quinoa, amaranth) require further investigation, however, so far the evidence confirms that they are as nutritious as modern varieties, maybe even more so.

A European Food Safety Authority report states that three servings per day of wholegrain (e.g. three slices of wholemeal bread or a portion of wholegrain rice, pasta or quinoa) can improve digestion function and gut health, help weight management, balance glucose and insulin levels and promote favourable cholesterol levels.

Although people in the UK tend to consume low amounts of wholegrain (20g/day compared to 55g/day in Denmark), there is currently no advice on the recommended intake. However, the 2015-2020 Dietary Guidelines for Americans recommends that at least half of one's grain intake should come from wholegrains.

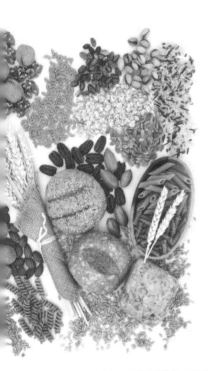

▶ Include three portions of wholegrains in your daily diet

▶ Choose products where the wholegrain ingredient is listed first on the label

▶ Start the day with porridge instead of a sugary cereal

Tip #26

Information

Choosing more wholegrains
Heart UK - https://go22.uk/wgservings
Includes a table of foods and the amount needed to provide one whole grain serving

Whole grain components, disease impacts and digestive health - Harvard School of Public Health
https://go22.uk/wholegrains

Retailers

Healthy Supplies - https://go22.uk/healthysup
Wide range of complete, rolled, powdered and puffed wholegrains

Is whole grain intake associated w/ reduced total & cause-specific death rates in older women?
American Journal of Public Health - https://go22.uk/rp0181
Total mortality risk was inversely associated with whole grain intake

Whole grain, bran, and germ intake and risk of type 2 diabetes
PLoS Medicine - https://go22.uk/rp0182
Whole grain intake is inversely associated with risk of type 2 diabetes

COST: ● ● ● ● ●   EASE: ● ● ● ● ●   IMPACT: ● ● ● ● ●

Air pollution in your area

Air pollution is associated with adverse health effects. For example, particulate air pollution is related to lung cancer and other cardiopulmonary mortality and cardiovascular diseases.

Air quality regulations can reduce air pollution at a societal level. For example, a ban on coal sales in Dublin, in 1990, led to a 70% reduction in black smoke within seventy-two months, and deaths from cardiovascular causes decreased significantly, by 10 % (243 fewer deaths/year) in this period.

London is considered the worst European capital regarding air quality. Not surprisingly, other places in the UK with poor air to breath are also cities, including Birmingham, Cardiff, Glasgow, Leeds and Manchester. Whilst the north and Cornwall have the best air quality in England, the Scottish Highlands have the cleanest air in the UK.

Studies indicate that living in highly polluted regions over several years increases cardiovascular morbidity and mortality, so it's important to reduce personal exposure by living in an area with better air quality. Air pollution may be only one thing being considered when picking the right location to live, along with work commitments and family connections, however, even within one town there is considerable variation in air quality. Pollution in one street may be half of that in another so it is worth putting in a put a bit of extra research for your long-term health.

Tip #27

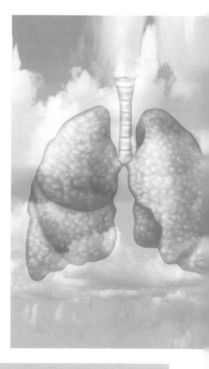

▶ Use an air quality map to pick a low pollution location to live

▶ During high air pollution days stay indoors as much as possible

▶ Campaign for improved air quality in your area/country

Information

World Air Quality Index (AQI) - https://go22.uk/waqi
Real-time air quality for more than10,000 stations

UK National Atmospheric Emissions Inventory key pollutant emission maps - https://go22.uk/naei

What is the Daily Air Quality Index?
DEFRA - https://go22.uk/daqi

Products

Flow personal air quality tracker - £129 (US$139)
Plume Labs - https://go22.uk/plumelabs
Measures concentration of NO2, VOC, PM2.5, PM10

Reduction in Fine Particulate Air Pollution and Mortality
American Journal of Respiratory and Critical Care Medicine - https://go22.uk/rp0191
Reduced PM2.5 concentrations were associated with reduced mortality risk

Effect of air-pollution control on death rates in Dublin, Ireland: an intervention study
Lancet - https://go22.uk/rp0192
Control of particulate air pollution could substantially diminish daily death

COST: ●●●● ○　　　EASE: ●●●● ○　　　IMPACT: ●● ○ ○ ○

Carbon monoxide

Carbon monoxide (CO) is a colourless, odourless, and toxic gas that is released from the incomplete burning of carbon-based fuels, such as wood, gas, and coal. In the absence of proper ventilation, CO is unable to escape and dangerous amounts of CO can accumulate indoors.

As well as faulty appliances, such as boilers and fires, deaths are regularly reported for campers and backyard BBQ chefs, who have the cooking too close to the tent or house to keep it out of the rain.

CO can kill within minutes and before its victims even know that CO is present. Unfortunately, this silent killer takes fifty lives every year in the UK. If CO enters your body, it replaces oxygen in your blood, meaning less oxygen reaches your heart, brain, and other vital organs.

Early symptoms of CO poisoning include breathing difficulties, headache, and fatigue. In severe cases, paralysis, brain damage and heart attacks can be caused as a result of prolonged exposure to CO. Although CO poisoning can be reversed if caught in time, it may reduce life expectancy and cause many long-term health problems such as neurological damage.

Being undetectable by humans, the only way to be warned of accumulating carbon monoxide is through the installation of an audible alarm.

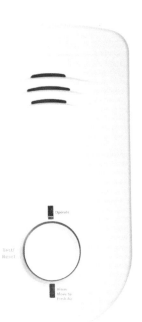

▶ Install a carbon monoxide detector in your home (and check it regularly)
▶ Don't bring your BBQ or camping stove inside
▶ Never leave a car idling, or run a generator, in an enclosed space

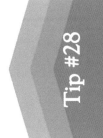

Tip #28

Information
Carbon Monoxide (CO) Poisoning Prevention
Centers for Disease Control and Prevention - https://go22.uk/coprevent

Products
Nest Protect - £109 (~US$140) - https://go22.uk/nest
Combined smoke and CO alarm with connectivity

FireAngel - £21-49 (~US$25-65) - https://go22.uk/fireangel
Range of CO alarms with alternative warning methods (strobe, vibrating pad) for the deaf

Long-term prognosis of patients with carbon monoxide poisoning: a nationwide cohort study
PLOS ONE - https://go22.uk/rp0511
Carbon monoxide poisoning significantly increases the long-term mortality risk.

Carbon Monoxide: From Awareness to Action
All-Party Parliamentary Carbon Monoxide Group - https://go22.uk/rp0512
The 92-page inquiry report warns that general public awareness-raising may be insufficient.

COST: ● ● ● ○ ○　　　　EASE: ● ● ● ● ○　　　IMPACT: ● ● ● ○ ○

Fire safety

According to the UK Fire & Rescue Services, 80% of fire-related fatalities occur in the home and only 20% in non-domestic buildings. A proactive approach will reduce your risk of a fire, and in the worst-case scenario, improve your chances of survival.

Correctly using appliances, safely cooking, smoking and heating is essential, as the major causes of home fires are related to smokers' materials (37%), cooking hazards (25%), improper heating, defective electrical systems and appliances. Fire detection and knowing your escape routes are also important, as US Fire Administration statistics show that 37% of fire victims in residential buildings were trying to escape, and 31% of victims were sleeping.

Fire deaths can generally be avoided by applying a safety toolkit to the home. First, install fire and smoke alarms, as in 50 % of UK domestic fires there was no operational smoke alarm. Keep in mind that inhaling toxic fumes is the primary cause of death in fires. Then buy a fire extinguisher (and a fire blanket for the kitchen) and learn how to use it. Make sure to have an escape plan and that all family members know it. If there is a risk of getting trapped upstairs, then invest in a fire ladder.

If a fire starts, get out the building. Leave behind your possessions. Stay out and yell "Fire!" in order to warn others. Call for the fire service.

Tip #29

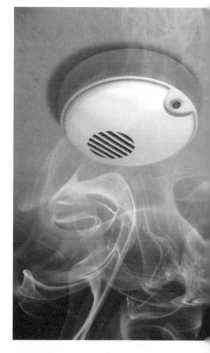

▶ **Install smoke alarms and check them regularly**

▶ **Involve all family members in setting up a fire escape plan**

▶ **Buy fire equipment, e.g. extinguishers, blankets and emergency ladders**

Information
Make your home safe from fire
UK Home Office - https://go22.uk/fire

Types of smoke alarms and where to fit them
UK Fire Service - https://go22.uk/smokealarms

Retailers
Safelincs - https://go22.uk/safelincs
Provides fire safety products and services to businesses, public bodies and end customers

Detailed analysis of fires attended by fire and rescue services in England
UK Home Office - https://go22.uk/rp0521

U.S. fire deaths, fire death rates, and risk of dying in a fire
U.S. Fire Administration - https://go22.uk/rp0522

COST: ● ● ● ● ●   EASE: ● ● ● ● ●   IMPACT: ● ● ● ○ ○

Fresh air and sunlight

The "Open Air Factor" (OAF) is a mixture of chemical agents that kills dangerous microorganisms and was first discovered by the UK military's chemical and biological research centre - it's also known as fresh air! The specific complex (produced by ozone-alkene reactions) is particularly common in rural air, and is not dangerous for humans since it is neutralized by our cells.

OAF has a very unstable nature, and can be extremely difficult to manipulate and characterize. However, it is known to be a naturally occurring germicidal agent, useful against several pathogenic microorganisms such as E. coli, S. epidermis, P. tularensis and others. It disappears very quickly in enclosed spaces and its antimicrobial effects work only on surfaces.

Sunlight is another factor found outdoors that brings its own benefits. It contains ultraviolet radiation, which is frequently used in sterile environments as a way to kill most microorganisms directly exposed to it. This explains why food contamination and some infections become more frequent or severe environments where ventilation is poor and there is no natural light source.

It is very important to clarify that although OAF is useful, there are many bacteria and other microorganisms that are resistant to it, for example, gram negative bacteria tend to be not very affected by it.

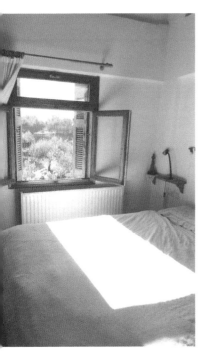

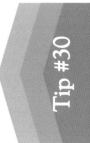

▷ Keep your home well ventilated with a window open whenever possible
▷ Keep curtains open during the day
▷ Leave a window slightly open in your bedroom at night

Tip #30

Information
The Open Air Factor
The Institute of Materials, Minerals and Mining - https://go22.uk/oafimmm
A story of OAFs and SODs, sausages and circumstances

Products
Air Vaccine 015+ Air Disinfection - £465 (US$599)
Aviva Natural Health Solutions - https://go22.uk/aviva015
Produces hydroxyl radicals to clean spaces for 100 – 1000 sq ft.

The germicidal effect of the open air in different parts of The Netherlands
The Journal of Hygiene - https://go22.uk/rp0601
Presence of bactericidal compounds could be demonstrated

Effect of ozone and open air factor against aerosolized Micrococcus luteus
Journal of Food Protection - https://go22.uk/rp0602
OAF is potentially an effective antibacterial agent that can reduce the microbial load in air

COST: ●●●●● EASE: ●●●●● IMPACT: ●●●●●

Indoor air pollution

Air pollution is generally thought of as something that only occurs outside. In fact, indoor air pollution is one of the top ten causes of death in the world. This undercover killer contributes to 4.3 million deaths worldwide, annually, according to WHO.

The truth is that the air in homes and workplaces can be more polluted than outdoor air. Pollutants include cooking fumes, dust, perfume, furniture, varnish, volatile organic chemicals (VOCs) and cigarette smoke. Our four-legged friends make it even worse.

Particulate matter (PM2.5) is the main villain here – this is fine particles smaller than 2.5 m wide - that's less than a hundredth of a millimeter. It derives from outdoor air and indoor sources. These tiny killers cause many respiratory and cardiovascular problems, including pneumonia, heart attacks and cancers. PM2.5 is the 13th leading cause of death worldwide. It contributes to about 800,000 premature deaths each year, according to the WHO.

Fortunately, indoor air pollution can be reduced by good quality air purifiers and the effects are almost immediate. For example, a study in Shangai found that using air filters for just forty-eight hours reduced the concentration of PM2.5 by 57%, with residents benefiting from a 3% lowering in blood pressure.

It's important that products are fitted with filters that can remove PM2.5 particles – typically this means using a HEPA filter. Ideally it should also have an activated carbon air filter to remove VOCs.

Tip #31

▷ Install an air purifier/filter where you spend most of your time

▷ Make sure it contains a HEPA filter and is rated to remove PM2.5

▷ Don't use an open fire or wood burner in your home

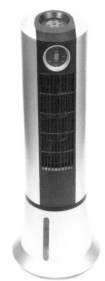

Products

Blueair air purifiers and monitors -
https://go22.uk/blueair
Prices range from £129 - £499 (US$169-649)

Dyson Pure Cool purifying desk fan - £399 (US$519)
https://go22.uk/dyson
Also comes in tower version with a heater.

Information

TIME magazine: Can Indoor Plants Really Purify the Air? - https://go22.uk/plants
Unfortunately, it seems only in laboratory conditions.

Evaluating the Long-Term Health and Economic Impacts of Central Residential Air Filtration
International Journal of Environmental Research and Public Health - https://go22.uk/rp0201
High-efficiency particle air filtration can reduce premature deaths and increase life expectancy.

Effects of Indoor Particles on Blood Pressure and Heart Rate among Young Adults in Taipei
Indoor Air - https://go22.uk/rp0202
Indoor PM10 and PM2.5 exposure was associated with an elevation in SBP, DBP, and HR.

COST: ● ● ● ○ ○   EASE: ● ● ● ○ ○   IMPACT: ● ● ○ ○ ○

Radon exposure

Radon is a chemically inert, colourless, odourless, gas that is also radioactive. It is common in nature and is formed underground (particularly in granite rock) and can seep into buildings through the floor.

Exposure to radon is the second leading cause of lung cancer in the United States, after smoking. Additionally, the effects of radon are exacerbated in smokers. If a person smokes and also lives in a house with high radon levels, the risk of developing lung cancer is especially high.

Studies indicate that children may be more sensitive to radon exposure because of their higher respiration rate and rapidly dividing cells, which are more vulnerable to radiation damage. Underground miners exposed to high levels of radon also have an excess risk of lung cancer.

Radon levels vary geographically, as its presence depends on the type of rock and soil composition. Radon can get into any types of buildings and represents a particular risk in homes where people spend more time and therefore are most likely to receive a greater exposure.

Radon testing methods are inexpensive (about £50/US$65) and are a useful way of assessing radon exposure at home. If the result is above the UK Action Level (200 Bq m-3) then steps to remedy the problem usually cost a few hundred pounds.

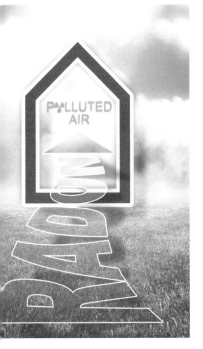

▷ Get your property tested if you live in a high radon area

▷ Take remedial action if test is positive (e.g. install a vent, fan or sump)

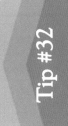

Tip #32

Information
Is your property in a radon Affected Area?
Radon map provided by Public Health England (PHE) - https://go22.uk/radonmap
Plus information for householders and those buying or selling a house

Five facts every home owner should know about radon
Public Health England - https://go22.uk/radonfacts

Residential radon and risk of lung cancer: a combined analysis of 7 studies
Epidemiology - https://go22.uk/rp0221
Direct evidence of an association between residential radon and lung cancer risk

Radon in homes and risk of lung cancer: analysis of 13 European case-control studies
BMJ - https://go22.uk/rp0222
Radon responsible for about 2% of all deaths from cancer in Europe

COST: ●●●○○   EASE: ●●●○○   IMPACT: ●●●○○

Trees

It's no secret that trees are one of nature's many wonders. Not only do trees provide a lovely look and fresh oxygen, but they also offer a cost-effective way to tackle urban air pollution. They act as natural air filters that trap pollutants from the air. Scientific research shows that the average reduction of particulate matter near trees is between 7-24%.

Trees can do wonders for health. Living near trees helps lengthen healthspan and reduce mortality rates. A recent study suggests that every ten trees in a block is equivalent to an increase of seven years of healthy life. Trees also help lower the risk of cardiovascular, respiratory and various metabolic diseases.

What's more, scientific research proves that green spaces improve recovery from surgery and boost the immune system. In addition, those living close to green spaces have improved mental well-being. Finally, leafy streets also help enhance recovery from stress and depressive disorders.

So, whether searching for an apartment to rent, or looking to buy a house, it's worth counting the number of trees in the location.

Tip #33

▶ Choose an apartment or a house in neighbourhoods with a higher density of trees
▶ Plant trees in your own garden or buy small ones for inside your home

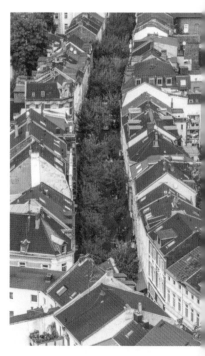

Organisations
Trees for Cities - https://go22.uk/trees4cities
UK charity working at a national and international scale to improve lives by creating greener cities

Woodland Trust - https://go22.uk/woodland
Over the next 10 years, we're aiming to plant 64 million trees and we can't do it without you

Information
Top trees for small gardens
Gardeners' World - https://go22.uk/toptrees

Residential green spaces and mortality: A systematic review
Environment International - https://go22.uk/rp0211
Living in areas with higher amounts of green spaces reduces all-cause and CVD mortality

The effect of urban green on small-area (healthy) life expectancy
J Epidemiol Community Health - https://go22.uk/rp0212
Both quantity and quality of urban green are related to increased life expectancy and healthspan

COST: ● ● ● ● ●   EASE: ● ● ● ● ○   IMPACT: ● ● ○ ○ ○

Dangerous sports

When deciding whether to take up (or continue) a particular activity, it's good to look at the chance of dying each time it is undertaken. BASE jumping has the worst mortality rate – one fatality in every 2,300 jumps which is much worse than one in every 100,000 parachute jumps. Scuba diving is twice as safe as parachuting (one death per 200,000 dives) and rock climbing deaths are about one in 320,000 climbs. For ski and snowboard lovers the risk is minimal – only one death per 1.5 million visits.

If anyone has enough money to be considering the upcoming space tourism flights, remember that an astronaut has around a one in sixty-two chance of dying on a mission. For reference, the odds of dying in a plane crash are one for every eleven million flights taken.

There are plenty of benefits to be gained from some of these activities, such as exercise and social relationships, so if you do decide to take part then respect some general rules: follow the training guidelines, know your limits and wear adequate equipment and clothing. Protective gear and clothing can be the difference between life and death.

Be particularly careful when enjoying something new on vacation – many traumatic deaths happen on holiday, outside the person's country of dwelling.

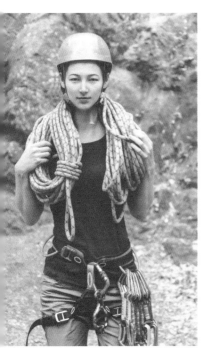

▶ Avoid sports with a high mortality rate

▶ Know the risks, know your limits

▶ Use appropriate safety equipment and make sure it is certified

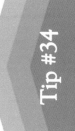

Tip #34

Information
Which Helmet for Which Activity?
US Consumer Product Safety Commission -
https://go22.uk/whichhelmet
List of activities and applicable standards

Buying and sizing a ski or snowboard helmet
Ski Club of Great Britain - https://go22.uk/skihelmets

Injuries in extreme sports
Journal of Orthopaedic Surgery and Research - https://go22.uk/skiinjuries
Appropriate safety gear is essential for protection from severe or fatal injuries as the margins for error in these sports are small.

Current Standards for Sports and Automotive Helmets: A Review
HEADS Innovation Training Network - https://go22.uk/helmets

COST: ● ● ● ● ●   EASE: ● ● ● ● ●   IMPACT: ● ● ○ ○ ○

Dental health

For most people, the need to maintain oral hygiene is driven by a desire for a nice smile and fresh breath, however dental health is also a factor in one's life expectancy. Surprisingly, poor oral health increases the risk of all-cause mortality and poses adverse effects on health outcomes.

Negligence towards oral hygiene leads to the development of oral diseases, such as dental caries, periodontal disease, dental erosion and tooth loss. These further pave the way for fatal diseases such as heart disease, diabetes, strokes and pneumonia. Evidence suggests that people with poor oral health are at a significantly higher risk of developing cardiovascular disease and respiratory diseases, especially if combined with smoking habits.

The reason for the association is the fact that unclean oral cavities house various harmful bacteria which find their way into the body and cause infection. Smoking also leads to gum disease because of the accumulation of bacterial plaque and in the worse cases can cause mouth cancer.

Oral health care also plays a vital role, during pregnancy, in preventing premature birth, low birth weight and pregnancy tumours (oral swelling). Pregnant women are at a higher risk of tooth decay and, hence, should keep their dental hygiene under check.

Tip #35

▶ Brush your teeth twice a day
▶ Floss daily (before cleaning your teeth)
▶ Have regular dental check-ups

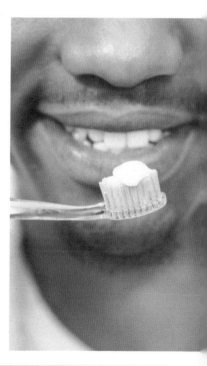

Organisations
Oral Health Foundation - https://go22.uk/ohf
Independent charity dedicated to improving oral health and wellbeing around the world.

Information
How to keep your teeth clean - https://go22.uk/teeth
NHS advice on toothbrushes, toothpaste & flossing

Products
Brush DJ - Free - https://go22.uk/brushdj
Plays 2 minutes of your music so you brush your teeth for the right amount of time

Relationship between oral health and mortality rate
Journal of Clinical Periodontology - https://go22.uk/rp0061
Poor oral health increases the risk of mortality especially for smokers

The prevalence and incidence of coronary heart disease is significantly increased in periodontitis
American Heart Journal - https://go22.uk/rp0062
Both the prevalence and incidence of CHD are significantly increased in PD

COST: ● ● ● ● ○   EASE: ● ● ● ● ○   IMPACT: ● ● ● ● ○

Exercise - aerobic

Aerobic exercise (or cardio training) can not only improve fitness but also extend lifespan. These activities cause your heart to pump extra oxygen rich blood to the muscles as a fuel, so both heart and breathing rate increase throughout the session.

As well as that, aerobic training increases stress in the body. This forces the body to adapt to it, becoming stronger and more prepared for new stress. These processes are positive because they activate pathways that act against inflammation which protects from chronic diseases.

Large epidemiological studies have confirmed that aerobic exercise can lower (by around a third) the incidence of heart disease, diabetes, and your general mortality rate. In practice, this leads to an increase of several years in life expectancy.

Aerobic exercise includes fast walking, running, jogging, swimming, rowing and cycling, and for people who prefer doing exercise indoors, gyms offer a range of different classes (such as step, BodyPump and Zumba) as well as stationary running and cycling machines. Team players also get an aerobic workout in fast-moving sports such as soccer, netball and basketball.

To save money, there are plenty of videos available on how to exercise at home.

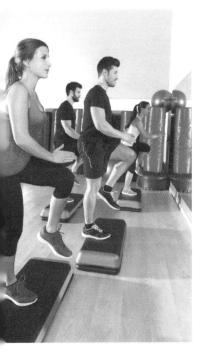

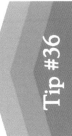

▷ Do at least 150 minutes of moderate-intensity aerobic activity every week
▷ Pick an activity that you enjoy to keep you motivated

Tip #36

Information
10-minute home cardio workout
NHS - https://go22.uk/10cardio
No equipment required

Products
Best fitness tracker 2018 - £25-169 (~US$32-218)
TechRadar's top 10 activity bands -
https://go22.uk/trackers2018

Does Physical Activity Increase Life Expectancy?
Journal of Aging Research - https://go22.uk/rp0891
All-cause mortality is decreased by about 30% to 35% in physically active subjects

Exercise Type and Intensity in Relation to Coronary Heart Disease in Men
JAMA - https://go22.uk/rp0892
Running for one or more hours per week was associated with a 42% risk reduction

COST: ● ● ● ● ●   EASE: ● ● ● ● ○   IMPACT: ● ● ○ ○ ○

Exercise - too much running

Can you have too much of a good thing? With running, it appears you can. Regular physical activity lowers the chance of developing respiratory and cardiovascular diseases, osteoporosis and some cancers. However, some research evidence warns that too much running may be bad as not running at all.

In one study of nearly 4,000 runners, two thirds of whom ran more than twenty miles a week, a decreased longevity was observed in the high mileage runners. However, this was not linked to any heart disease factors and the underlying cause of the U-shaped relationship between training distance and longevity remains unclear.

So, what is the optimal exercise level that provides the highest health benefit? Current recommendations suggest at least seventy-five minutes of vigorous-intensity or 150 minutes of moderate-intensity aerobic activity per week. Epidemiological data shows that it's best to run no more than twenty miles per week at seven miles per hour to maximise lifespan. If your exercise is exclusively running then these two recommendations may contradict, so to avoid that it is better incorporate a mix of aerobic and weight-training activities into your programme. Also, the weekly mileage allowance shouldn't all be done in a single session.

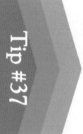

Tip #37

▶ Avoid regularly running twenty miles per week at a fast pace

▶ Run for no more than one hour in one session

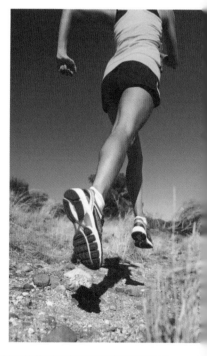

Information
Too Much Running Tied to Shorter Life Span
WebMD - https://go22.uk/runspan

Can Too Much Exercise Harm the Heart?
The New York Times - https://go22.uk/harmheart

Products
MapMyRun – https://go22.uk/mapmyrun
App to map routes and track activity. Free.

Are CVD risk factors responsible for the u-shaped relationship between running and longevity?
Journal of the American College of Cardiology - https://go22.uk/rp0771
Those who ran >20 miles per week did not experience a longer lifespan vs non-runners

Exercise and the heart: The good, the bad, and the ugly
European Heart Journal - https://go22.uk/rp0772
Vigorous endurance exercise is associated with arrhythmias, myocardial fibrosis, possibly CAD

COST: ● ● ● ○ ○   EASE: ● ● ● ○ ○   IMPACT: ● ● ● ○ ○

Exercise - weight lifting

As people grow older, they become weaker. They lose the strength in their muscles and bones, which causes problems with mobility and limits everyday activities. This weakening can be combatted with weightlifting or other strength training exercises even, and especially, in the elderly. Importantly, scientific papers also found that strength exercises can prolong lifespan by increasing and maintaining lean muscle mass.

Strength exercises can help in weight management and lower the risk of heart disease and diabetes. In a recent study, people with a good grip strength when 65 to 74 years old lived five years longer than those with weak strength.

Weight training isn't only about lifting weights, curling dumbbells and doing bench presses in the gym. It can also be done at home with resistance bands or by using one's own body weight, for example press ups (push ups), squats and sit-ups.

Whichever way it is done, muscle strengthening exercise is all about quality, not quantity. One exercise set should involve eight to twelve repetitions, with sufficient weight that it would be a struggle to complete another repetition. Older exercisers may prefer to lift lighter weights and do more repetitions to reduce pressure on the joints.

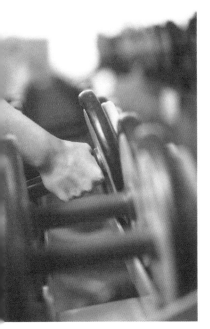

▶ Perform muscle-strengthening activities twice a week

▶ Target all major muscle groups (legs, hips, back, abdomen, chest, shoulders and arms)

Tip #38

Information
NHS strength exercises - https://go22.uk/strengthex
Gentle and easy to follow strength exercise routine that can be done at home

People with Low Muscle Strength More Likely to Die Prematurely
University of Michigan - https://go22.uk/strengthdie

Products
Best weightlifting apps
Digital Trends - https://go22.uk/weightapps
iOS and Android apps that include instruction videos, workout plans and exercise logs

Strength Training and All-Cause, Cardiovascular Disease, and Cancer Mortality in Older Women
Journal of the American Heart Association - https://go22.uk/rp0941
A moderate amount of time in strength training seemed beneficial for longevity

Exercise Type and Intensity in Relation to Coronary Heart Disease in Men
JAMA - https://go22.uk/rp0942
Weight training is associated with reduced risk of coronary heart disease

COST: ● ● ● ● ●   EASE: ● ● ● ● ●   IMPACT: ● ● ○ ○ ○

Hand hygiene

Good hand hygiene provides protection against many potentially deadly diseases. Respiratory viruses and gastrointestinal illnesses are very common health risks accounting for about 10% of all deaths in the EU. They frequently attack vulnerable individuals, such as young children or older adults. The causes of these conditions can be found in many things we touch including water, food and most surfaces, therefore, reducing our exposure is important for prevention.

There are plenty of options for maintaining good hand hygiene. Many different products claim to help prevent diseases by killing bacteria and viruses, however, it is known within the scientific community that under normal conditions "antibacterial" soap or gels are no more effective than plain soap in removing pathogens from skin. Alcohol-based products tend to be recommended as an alternative in low-income settings.

The effectiveness of hand hygiene against different diseases depends on several factors including: daily routine, the product used, frequency of use, and surrounding environment, among others. People in a high-risk environment should follow a more strict and in-depth cleaning protocol.

Tip #39

▶ Wash your hands at least twice per day with soap and water
▶ Wash your hands before cooking or touching your mouth
▶ Wash thoroughly, including between, and ends of, fingers

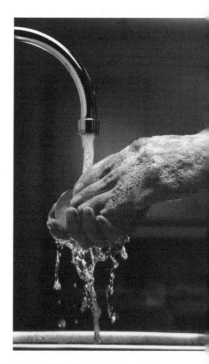

Information
How to wash your hands (video)
NHS - https://go22.uk/washhands
Washing your hands properly should take about as long as singing "Happy Birthday" twice (around twenty seconds)

Show Me the Science - Situations where hand sanitizer can be effective
Centers for Disease Control and Prevention - https://go22.uk/sanitizer

Effect of Hand Hygiene on Infectious Disease Risk in the Community Setting: A Meta-Analysis
American Journal of Public Health (AJPH) - https://go22.uk/rp1101
Improvements in hand hygiene resulted in reductions in gastrointestinal and respiratory illness. Use of antibacterial soap showed little added benefit compared with nonantibacterial soap.

COST: ●●●● ○   EASE: ●●●● ○   IMPACT: ●●● ○ ○

Reading

It is widely known that sustained low activity levels and lack of movement leads to reduced life expectancy and health problems. However, and conversely, recent studies suggest that frequent engagement in sedentary leisure activities, such as reading novels, playing card games or handcrafting may increase longevity.

A study conducted by the Hadassah Hebrew University from Israel, in 2008, was the first to propose that reading habits had a positive effect on longevity. Stockholm University later confirmed this in a study of 1,246 men and women aged over 65 years old, confirming that the benefits on life expectancy of reading books apply to both genders.

In 2016, a large-scale study, conducted by Yale University, replicated and extended these results on adults over 50 years old. The findings highlighted that, regardless of the participants' gender, wealth, education, or health, reading books was associated with a 20% reduction in risk of mortality. Importantly, they found that the benefit of reading books was significantly higher than that observed for reading newspapers or magazines.

Furthermore, the benefits of reading books may also improve quality of life in the elderly. Indeed, the literature suggests that spending between four to six hours a week reading books not only reduces the risk of incident dementia but also lowers the probability of developing Alzheimer's Disease.

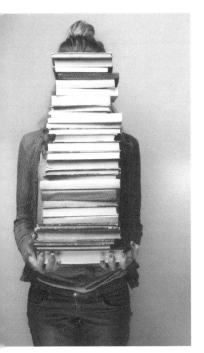

▷ Take time to read a proper book – rather than short articles

▷ Find a reading partner or join a book group

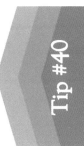

Tip #40

Information
6 Practical Tips to Help Cultivate a Reading Habit
Huffington Post - https://go22.uk/readingtips

Products
ReadPrint (free) - https://go22.uk/readprint
Offers thousands of free books, from Shakespeare pieces to science fiction stories

Good Reads (free) - https://go22.uk/goodreads
World's largest site for readers and book recommendations. Track the books you're reading and share with your friends.

A chapter a day: Association of book reading with longevity
Social Science & Medicine - https://go22.uk/rp0551
Book readers experienced a 20% reduction in risk of mortality over a twelve-year-period

Engagement in Reading and Hobbies and Risk of Incident Dementia
American Journal of Alzheimer's Disease & Other Dementias - https://go22.uk/rp0552
Hobbies for one or more hours every day might be protective against dementia in late life

COST: ●●●●●   EASE: ●●●● ○   IMPACT: ●●●● ○

Recreational drugs

There is an interesting trend in Europe and the UK. Recently, adults from 40 to 50 years old have become the age group with the highest risk of accidental death through the abuse of recreational drugs. Heroin, cocaine, amphetamines and MDMA (ecstasy) are the most popular in this group. Interestingly, chronic use is not a common requirement associated with death, meaning that even new users are in danger.

There are many ways in which a person can die from drug abuse; most of them are accidental (e.g. overdose, incorrect administration, contamination) or because of irresponsible behaviour while under their influence (e.g. car crashes) rather than because of their biological toxicity.

The deadliest drug is heroin, followed by amphetamines and cocaine. Someone using several drugs will be more vulnerable than those only using one.

Ecstasy and marijuana may be regarded as "soft drugs," and are statistically less deadly than most other drugs, however, they still increase the risk of dying by up to five times the normal average. The chance of dying for first time ecstasy users is estimated to be somewhere between the risk of dying in a base jump (parachuting off a building or cliff) and a single skydive.

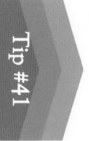

Tip #41

▶ Avoid using any recreational drugs –
and definitely don't mix them

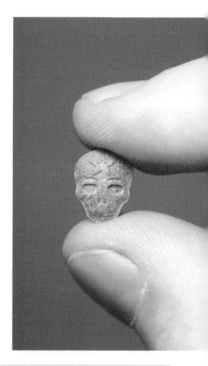

Information
The effects of drugs
NHS - https://go22.uk/nhsdrugs
Health-focused information about common drugs and their impacts.

Coming off drugs
The Mix - https://go22.uk/offdrugs
Guide to cleaning up safely - whatever drug you're dependent on.

The Loop - https://go22.uk/theloop
Provides drug safety testing, welfare and harm reduction services at nightclubs and festivals

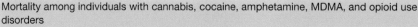

Mortality among individuals with cannabis, cocaine, amphetamine, MDMA, and opioid use disorders
Drug and alcohol dependence - https://go22.uk/rp1031
Results revealed different mortality ratios for different drugs

Review of deaths related to taking ecstasy, England and Wales, 19977-2000
BMJ - https://go22.uk/rp1032

COST: ●● ● ● ●   EASE: ●●● ● ●   IMPACT: ●●● ● ●

Saunas

Dry saunas are designed to heat up the body using temperatures around 90 °C (190 °F) and humidity below 20%, and have been associated with increased longevity. The reasoning behind this claim is that the lowering of blood pressure and enhancement of ventricular function that comes from the frequent use of saunas can bring benefits for those with cardiovascular disease.

In 2015, a Finnish study reported an up to 18% decreased mortality among middle-aged men, with cardiovascular disease, who used saunas between four to seven times per week compared with people who used saunas only once a week.

As an added benefit, the dry air can help some patients with psoriasis, who report relief from itching. In addition, asthmatics may experience less wheezing.

Although jumping into an ice bath or getting under a cold-water pail following a sauna are popular practices in some cultures, it is best to cool down slowly to prevent circulatory stress which could negate all the benefits.

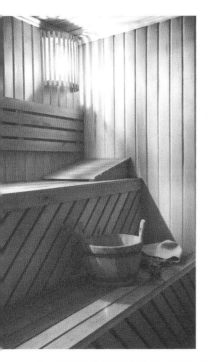

▶ Enjoy a sauna at least once a week
▶ Cool down gradually afterward
▶ People with existing heart conditions should check with their doctor before using saunas

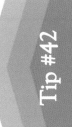
Tip #42

Information

Sauna Health Benefits
Harvard Medical School - https://go22.uk/saunaben
A sauna benefits your heart health, as long as you practice sauna safety

Do infrared saunas have any health benefits?
Mayo Clinic - https://go22.uk/irsaunas

Products

21 Inexpensive Sauna and Hot Tub Design Ideas
Morning Chores - https://go22.uk/hottubideas
Links to how to build a sauna in your home or a shed, and even a portable bike sauna!

Association Between Sauna Bathing and Fatal Cardiovascular and All-Cause Mortality Events
JAMA Internal Medicine - https://go22.uk/rp0121
Sauna bathing is associated with a reduced risk cardiovascular death, and all-cause mortality

Clinical Effects of Regular Dry Sauna Bathing: A Systematic Review
Evidence-Based Complementary and Alternative Medicine - https://go22.uk/rp0122
Infrared and/or Finnish sauna bathing has potential to provide many beneficial health effects

COST: ● ● ● ● ●   EASE: ● ● ● ● ○   IMPACT: ● ● ● ● ○

Sedentary behaviour

Sedentary behaviour refers to routines lacking in physical activity and frequently leads to weight gain and more serious health problems that result in a lower life expectancy.

The correlation between sedentarism and poor health has been confirmed by many scientists throughout the decades, to the point where sedentarism is now seen as the main cause of many cardiovascular and metabolic diseases. Research has now migrated to the finer aspects of its impact on disease; for example, it was discovered that occupational sitting (i.e. at work) is less harmful than casual sitting (resting, gaming, watching TV, etc).

Daily routines with high amounts of physical activity (not necessarily exercise) can bring great benefits for the individual, both reducing mortality and increasing healthspan. But, it is important to note that intense, infrequent surges of physical activity ("weekend warriors") do not counteract the effects of long-term sedentary behaviour.

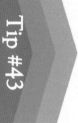

Tip #43

▶ Avoid sitting for more than five hours each day

▶ If you work at a desk, stand up and move around every thirty minutes

▶ Watch TV standing up

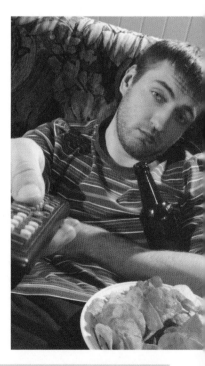

Information
What Sitting Down All Day Does To Your Body
Huffington Post - https://go22.uk/sittingdown
How It Affects The Spine, Organs And Circulation

Products
Massage Balls
Physio Room - https://go22.uk/massageballs
If you're unable to get up regularly, keep a pair of these nearby and keep your legs moving while giving yourself a foot massage

Sedentary behaviour and risk of mortality from all-causes & cardiometabolic diseases in adults
British Journal of Sports Medicine - https://go22.uk/rp0331
Total sitting time is associated with all cause and cardiometabolic disease-related mortality

Sedentary Behaviour and Physical Activity Are Independent Predictors of Successful Aging in Middle-Aged and Older Adults
Journal of Aging Research - https://go22.uk/rp0332

COST: ● ● ● ● ●   EASE: ● ● ● ● ○   IMPACT: ● ● ● ● ○

Sleep duration

Industrialised societies tend to dedicate more hours to work, watching television and using the internet, which leads to dramatic changes in sleep habits, and results in later sleep times and less sleep. For instance, in the United States, the average amount of sleep has decreased by around 20% over the past century.

Multiple studies suggest that lack of sleep leads to an increased risk of disease and mortality. More surprisingly perhaps, new research points out that more than eight hours of sleep also leads to increased risk of all-cause mortality (e.g. cancer-related and cardiovascular-related mortality). For instance, a study conducted on more than one million adults revealed that sleeping seven hours per night was sufficient to maximize survival, and sleeping more than eight hours or less than six hours per night showed an increased mortality risk – with the highest risk in those who slept less than four-and-a-half hours.

Sleeping pill use has often been associated to increased mortality, reaching 1.5 times the mortality rates of those who never used them. Most of the time sleeping pills are not necessary. Most people who complain of insomnia, or of waking during the night, have perfectly satisfactory sleep patterns, they just don't realise it.

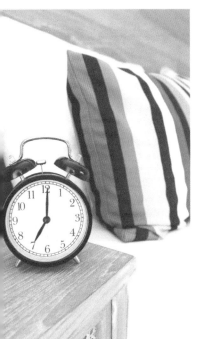

▶ **Aim to sleep around 7 hours per night**
▶ **Avoid using sleeping pills**

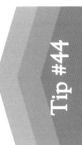

Tip #44

Information

Natural Sleep Aids and Remedies
WebMD - https://go22.uk/sleepaids
Discusses melatonin, valerian, chamomile and more

5 ways to sleep more soundly
Mayo Clinic - https://go22.uk/sleepsound

Products

The best sleep tracking tech 2018 -
https://go22.uk/sleeptrack
T3 reviews the Withings Aura Sleep System, ResMed S+ sleep tracking system and Zeeq's Smart Pillow

Nighttime sleep duration, 24-hour sleep duration and risk of all-cause mortality among adults
Scientific Reports - https://go22.uk/rp0031
7 hours/day of sleep should be recommended to prevent premature death among adults

Mortality Associated With Sleep Duration and Insomnia
JAMA Psychiatry - https://go22.uk/rp0032
Above 7.5 hours, the longer participants reported sleeping, the greater their mortality hazard

COST: ● ● ● ● ●   EASE: ● ● ● ● ◯   IMPACT: ● ◯ ◯ ◯ ◯

Sleep position

The way we sleep is just as important as the quality and duration of our snooze. A recent study suggests that body posture during sleep affects the risk of neurodegenerative diseases, memory loss, and other health problems.

The brain produces metabolic waste that needs to be removed. The accumulation of this metabolic waste harms nerve cells and forms plaques, a factor in developing many neurodegenerative diseases. The rest of the body uses the lymphatic system to kill microbes and clear out cellular debris, but that does not extend into the brain. Only in the last few years has a network of lymphatic vessels, called the meningeal lymphatic vascular system, been discovered that perform the same waste clearance function in the brain.

Research has also revealed that this waste pathway is most effective when people sleep on their side (in the lateral position) compared to sleeping on their back or face down. As an added bonus, it also reduces the occurrence of sleep apnea.

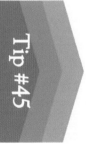

Tip #45

▶ Sleep on your side instead of on your back

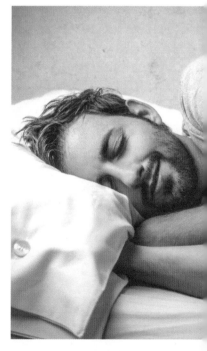

Information

Could Body Posture During Sleep Affect How Your Brain Clears Waste?
Stony Brook University -
https://go22.uk/sleepposture

Sleep Apnea and Sleeping Positions: Which is Best (or Worst)?
Eden Sleep - https://go22.uk/sleepapnea

The Effect of Body Posture on Brain Glymphatic Transport
Journal of Neuroscience - https://go22.uk/rp0611
Waste, including AB, removal was most efficient in the lateral position

Lateral sleeping position reduces severity of central sleep apnea / Cheyne-Stokes respiration
Sleep - https://go22.uk/rp0612
This effect is independent of postural effects on the upper airway

COST: ● ● ● ● ●   EASE: ● ○ ○ ○ ○   IMPACT: ● ● ● ● ●

Smoking

Smoking causes oral and lung cancer, respiratory and vascular diseases. There is a very clear correlation between the intensity of smoking and mortality risk, and on average, life expectancy is reduced by eight years for men and ten years for women compared to non-smokers.

The lethal effects of smoking are attributed to tobacco smoke which comprises 5,000 different chemicals. The bundle of these toxic and carcinogenic compounds claims the lives of 50% of its users which contribute to seven million deaths each year. Of these, nearly one million deaths are of non-smokers, which occur because of second-hand smoke. Passive smoking poses the same extent of threat to health as direct smoking.

Shisha cafes, where people inhale flavoured tobacco smoke after it has passed through a water basin, are becoming popular in the UK. But using a hookah pipe is no less harmful than smoking as the carcinogens still make it through the water. It may even be worse than cigarettes as the amount of smoke inhaled in a single puff of shisha can be the same as that from a whole cigarette.

The good news is, quitting smoking during the early thirties avoids more than 90% of the risks attributed to tobacco and improves the prospects of survival to a very similar level to that of non-smokers.

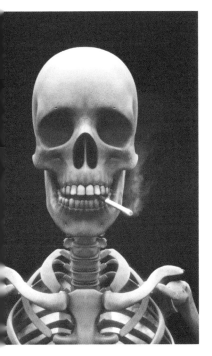

▶ DO NOT smoke

▶ Quit now, if you do

▶ Avoid areas where others are smoking

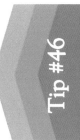

Tip #46

Information
10 health benefits of stopping smoking
NHS - https://go22.uk/nhssmoking
Including more energy, less stress and better sex

Free, proven support to help you quit!
NHS - https://go22.uk/nhsquit

Products
The Top 8 Products to Help You Quit Smoking
Healthline - https://go22.uk/quitsmoking
Including patches, gum and apps

Tobacco smoking and all-cause mortality in a large Australian cohort study
BMC Medicine - https://go22.uk/rp0231
Mortality risk increases with increasing smoking intensity

Smoking , smoking cessation, and lung cancer in the UK since 1950
BMJ - https://go22.uk/rp0232
People who quit smoking in middle-age avoid most subsequent risks attributed to tobacco

COST: ● ● ● ● ●   EASE: ● ● ● ○ ○   IMPACT: ● ● ○ ○ ○

Sunbeds

Tanning is the visible sign of skin damage. Ultraviolet (UV) rays penetrate deep into the skin and damage the DNA in its cells - in response to which, dark melanin pigments are produced. This damage can lead the cells to divide uncontrollably thereby leading to skin cancer, as well as premature ageing, wrinkles, and erythema. The impact of this harmful radiation varies depending on the strength of the UV rays, exposure time, frequency of use, skin type, and age.

It's a myth that sunbeds are a safe alternative to the sun – as both emit UV rays. Use of sunbeds by fair-skinned, younger individuals doubles the risk of developing skin cancers. In the UK, the use of sunbeds by the individuals under 18 years of age is prohibited by law.

Studies have also debunked some other common myths - indoor tanning does not cure acne (but may further complicate the situation) and doesn't provide protection from burning in the sun.

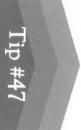

Tip #47

▸ Avoid sunbeds entirely
▸ Apply sunscreen 30 minutes before sun exposure and reapply regularly
▸ Check your skin regularly for signs of cancer

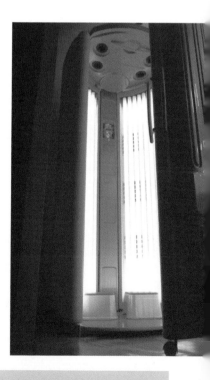

Information
Checking for skin cancer
SunSmart - https://go22.uk/sunsmart

Sunbeds and cancer
Cancer Research UK - https://go22.uk/sunbeds

Products
4 must-have gadgets & apps to stay safe in the sun
LifeWire - https://go22.uk/sungadgets

7 best fake tans
Independent - https://go22.uk/7faketans
NOTE: Fake tans do not protect against UV radiation

The epidemiology of UV induced skin cancer
Journal of Photochemistry and Photobiology B: Biology - https://go22.uk/rp0821
Risk increases with increasing ambient solar radiation

Cutaneous melanoma attributable to sunbed use: systematic review and meta-analysis
BMJ - https://go22.uk/rp0822
The use of sunbeds is associated with higher risk of occurrence of skin cancer

COST: ● ● ● ● ●   EASE: ● ● ● ● ○   IMPACT: ● ● ○ ○ ○

Tattoos

Tattooing has been practiced for thousands of years for decoration, to inflict punishment and to mark a status in society. Recently, tattoos have become more of a fashion trend with around half of all twenty-somethings having one – and almost one in four regretting it later.

Unfortunately, tattoos aren't a harmless adornment – there is a risk involved in the procedure, as well as from the ink itself.

The composition of tattoo inks is not regulated. Research suggests that the pigments are mainly organic pigments and heavy metal salts (coloured ink) some of which are carcinogenic. Some inks are loaded with high amounts of impurities and microbiological contamination which may prove detrimental to health. The US Food and Drug Administration regards most tattoo inks as more suitable for automobile paint than the skin.

Poor skin preparation or equipment sterilisation can result in staphylococcus aureus or pseudomonas bacteria infections. More seriously, having a tattoo risks a hepatitis C infection. Tattoo inks can also interfere with MRI scans making the diagnosis of a disease difficult and inaccurate.

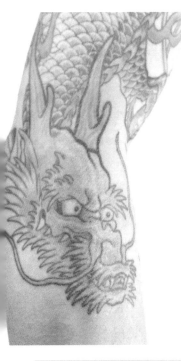

▷ They are low risk, but it's safer to avoid getting a tattoo

▷ If you must, then make sure you use a licensed and well-regarded artist

▷ If you have concerns about an existing tattoo, speak to a doctor

Tip #48

Information
Tattoos: Leaving their mark
Harvard Health Letter - https://go22.uk/tattoomark

Tattoo removal
NHS - https://go22.uk/removetat

Products
These Temporary Tattoo Brands Will Remedy Your Tat Fix, Without The Commitment
Huffington Post - https://go22.uk/temptats

Cutaneous complications related to permanent decorative tattooing
Expert Review of Clinical Immunology - https://go22.uk/rp0811
Primarily include infections, hypersensitivity, benign and sometimes malignant tumors

Tattooing and the risk of transmission of hepatitis C: a systematic review and meta-analysis
International Journal of Infectious Diseases - https://go22.uk/rp0812
Tattooing is associated with higher risk of Hepatitis C infection

COST: ●● ● ● ●   EASE: ●● ● ● ●   IMPACT: ●●● ● ●

Dog ownership

Dog ownership is found to have a positive effect on physical and mental well-being, resulting in an improved overall quality of life. Furthermore, studies have found that dog ownership is negatively associated with mortality, which means dog owners live longer.

Dog owners are shown to be at lower risk of developing cardiovascular disease and exhibit enhanced recovery from stroke, heart attack, and cancer. Ownership has also been associated with increased physical activity in adults and children.

Dog ownership has been accused of increased risk of allergic reactions, but studies indicate that it does not aggravate asthma, allergic rhinitis, or eczema. On the other hand, exposing infants to dogs in their first year of life can provide immune boosting benefits.

From the perspective of psychological well-being, dogs have been referred to as "social catalysts" as they increase contact with society. As their owner's companion, dogs influence their well-being by providing emotional support which protects the owner against anxiety related illness, stress and depression.

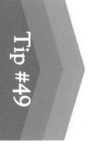

Tip #49

▶ Keep a dog as a pet (if you have enough room, time and money)

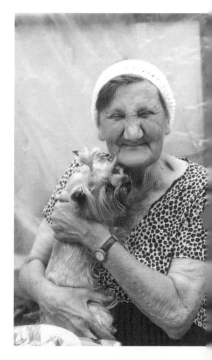

Information

How to look after and care for a dog – RSPCA
https://go22.uk/rspca
Including a downloadable leaflet and a guide to dogs and the law.

Simple steps for avoiding infections from dogs and cats - Harvard Health Blog
https://go22.uk/pets

Dog ownership and the risk of cardiovascular disease and death – a nationwide cohort study
Scientific Reports - https://go22.uk/rp0841
Dog ownership is associated with lower mortality and lower risk of cardiovascular disease.

Animal-assisted therapy at Mayo Clinic: The time is now
Complementary Therapies in Clinical Practice - https://go22.uk/rp0842
Heart attack patients who have a companion animal have a 5-fold increase in one-year survival.

COST: ● ● ● ● ●   EASE: ● ● ● ● ●   IMPACT: ● ● ○ ○ ○

Laughter

Laughter is the best medicine? Not quite, but it definitely has some benefits. Brain scans reveal that laughter triggers chemical responses, which lead to a sense of well-being and other research has shown that this translates to physical well-being too.

One study at the University of Texas, Austin, found artery function improved immediately after watching a humorous thirty-minute video (but decreased after watching a documentary) and this improvement lasted almost 24 hours.

In another study, laughter was associated with a significant increase in the activity of natural killer (NK) cells, which identify and kill cancerous cells (e.g. leukaemia, carcinomas, sarcomas and melanomas). However, this increase in NK cells only occurred in those subjects that actually laughed during exposure to a humorous stimulus, such as watching a comedy video, rather than just observing it.

Other studies have also found that it seems to be the physical action of laughing that counts, as in a recent study of ninety-one literary humourists and a matched group of serious authors it was the serious writers that lived longer.

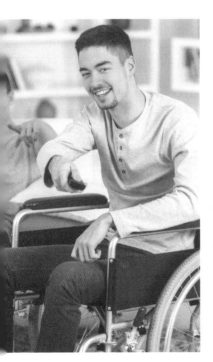

▷ Include activities to make you laugh every day – subscribe to a comic strip, watch your favourite sitcom, watch some YouTube antics

▷ Attend comedy events – stand-up, musicals, films

Tip #50

Information
Does Laughing Have Real Health Benefits?
Time Magazine - https://go22.uk/laughing

Products
The 25 Best Sunday Comic Strips of All Time
Complex - https://go22.uk/comics
The definitive collection including Garfield, Dilbert, Peanuts, The Far Side and Calvin and Hobbes.

The 20 Best TV Comedies of the 21st Century
Indiewire - https://go22.uk/comedies
Another great list including Peep Show, Scrubs, Sex and the City, and The Office.

15-Year Follow-Up Study of Sense of Humor and Causes of Mortality: Nord-Trøndelag
Psychosomatic Medicine - https://go22.uk/rp0561
Sense of humor is positively associated with survival from mortality related to CVD & infections

The effect of mirthful laughter on stress and natural killer cell activity
Alternative therapies in health and medicine - https://go22.uk/rp0562
Laughter is protective of cancer.

COST: ● ● ● ● ●   EASE: ● ● ● ○ ○   IMPACT: ● ● ● ○ ○

Meditation

People spend almost half of their waking hours thinking about something that is not related to what they are doing in that same moment. This fact has been revealed in a recent study conducted by psychologists at Harvard University. However, according to many philosophical and spiritual practices, "a wandering mind is an unhappy mind". Mindfulness and meditation try to overcome mind wandering – and there is evidence to suggest that these practices improve quality of life, health and longevity.

Since 1930, the effects of meditation practices on health and life expectancy have been extensively studied. More than 1500 studies have been conducted in the last century, suggesting that meditation and mindfulness-based interventions are linked to a wide range of benefits including lower heart rate, blood pressure and oxygen consumption, as well as decreased anxiety, stress and nervousness. These improvements have then been observed to reduce the incidence of cardiovascular disease in practitioners.

There are many different forms and schools of meditation, with various techniques that either focus the mind on a particular object or open it to be aware of thoughts and sensations. They can be practised either in private or in a group.

Tip #51

▶ **Aim to meditate for ten minutes every day**

▶ **Learn the basics of mindfulness**

▶ **Be mindful during daily routines such as cleaning your teeth**

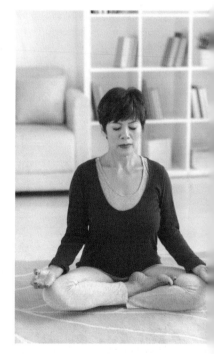

Information
How to Meditate
Harvard Medical School - https://go22.uk/meditate
Links for Guided Meditation Practice

Products
Free Mindfulness Project -
https://go22.uk/mindfulness
Over thirty free guided and self-guided audio exercises for download

Best Meditation Apps of 2018
Healthline - https://go22.uk/meditateapps

Review of Controlled Research: Transcendental Meditation Program & Cardiovascular Disease
Cardiology in Review - https://go22.uk/rp0091
Highly significant reduction in all-cause mortality, strong trend to reduction of CVD mortality

Meditation and blood pressure: a meta-analysis of randomized clinical trials
Journal of Hypertension - https://go22.uk/rp0092
Meditation may serve as a promising alternative approach for lowering both SBP and DBP

COST: ●●●○○   EASE: ●●●●○   IMPACT: ●●●●○

Relationships

A number of studies indicate that social support and inclusion may have a positive influence on life expectancy. Indeed, social isolation among seniors seems to be associated with a higher risk of depression, heart disease, and hypertension, even exceeding the risk associated with diabetes or smoking.

Surprisingly, social deficits are even more predictive of death in younger subjects than in those older than 65 years. Furthermore, these effects are related to measures of actual and perceived social isolation, even when these two measures do not necessarily correlate. For instance, during adolescence, perceived social isolation is significantly related to a high risk of obesity. As a consequence, it has a drastic impact on young metabolic and cardiovascular functioning, thus increasing the risk of premature death during adulthood.

The positive impact of forming and maintaining social connections operates at three different domains: behavioural, psychosocial and physiological. Behaviourally, being married or/and tied to religious organisations facilitates the formation of healthy habits and leads to lower risk of mortality. Psychologically, social support reduces stress and prevents depression. The physiological consequences of social inclusion have been widely supported by a number of studies, for example those suggesting a decreased susceptibility to the common cold and lower risk of more serious conditions, such as cancer, hypertension, and heart disease.

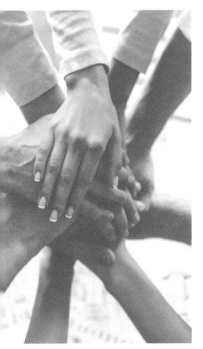

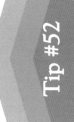

▷ Socialise with others at least once a week

▷ Invest time and effort in forming new social connections

▷ Join clubs, groups or societies in subjects that you are interested in

Tip #52

Information
101 Conversation Starters People Love
Tower of Power - https://go22.uk/conversation

Organisations
Meetup - https://go22.uk/meetup
Groups all around the world meeting up to discuss all things imaginable

Join an older people's group
Age UK - https://go22.uk/ageuk

Loneliness and Social Isolation as Risk Factors for Mortality: A Meta-Analytic Review
Perspectives on Psychological Science - https://go22.uk/rp0241
Both objective and subjective social isolation are predictive of death in 65 year-olds

Social Relationships and Mortality Risk: A Meta-analytic Review
PLOS Medicine - https://go22.uk/rp0242
Stronger social relationships had a 50% increased likelihood of survival

COST: EASE: IMPACT:

Speaking another language

The changes that occur in the brain upon speaking a second language have been show to improve its cognitive capacity. Research suggests that a stimulating environment, which includes learning new languages, makes the brain comparatively more resilient to the adverse effects of ageing or disease.

The benefits of being able to speak more than one language are not only restricted to social and professional benefits but further extend to the prevention of age-related cognitive decline.

Bilingualism has been shown to delay the onset of diseases related to cognitive impairment, such as dementia and Alzheimer's disease. Studies have also reported that bilinguals recover faster in terms of cognitive control after a stroke, which denotes an improved ability to cope with the damage to the brain.

The grey matter in our brains (which contains the cell bodies, dendrites and axon terminals of neurons) is critical for cognitive functions, such as memory and attention which tend to reduce with age. Bilinguals are found to have a greater volume of grey matter than monolinguals, which demonstrates the mental health benefits of speaking another language.

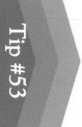

▶ If you only speak one language, learn to speak another

▶ Practice speaking a few words of more than one language every day

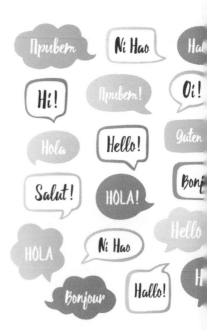

Information
The amazing benefits of being bilingual
BBC - https://go22.uk/bilingual

Products
Duolingo - https://go22.uk/duolingo
Thirty-two free courses. 2013 iPhone app of the year

BBC Languages - https://go22.uk/bbclanguages
Courses and phrases, audio and video, vocabulary, pronunciation, grammar, activities and tests

Bilingualism as a protection against the onset of symptoms of dementia
Neuropsychologia - https://go22.uk/rp0951
Bilingualism delays the onset of dementia

Impact of Bilingualism on Cognitive Outcome After Stroke
Stroke - https://go22.uk/rp0952
Bilinguals exhibited better cognitive outcome after stroke as compared to monolinguals

COST: ● ● ● ● ○   EASE: ● ● ○ ○ ○   IMPACT: ● ● ● ● ○

Stress

Stress is a complex subject. At a basic level there are two types of stress: acute (short term) and chronic (long term). Both have been studied for years and although much has been learned about how people process stress, there are still a lot of gaps in our understanding of exactly how stress affects behaviour and health.

Long- and short-term stress create somewhat similar reactions in the body. Chronic stress is simply a prolonged reaction to a persistent stressful situation, whatever that might be - disease in the family, overdue bills, or relationship issues. There is evidence linking chronic stress (high levels of cortisol during a long period of time) with lowered immune function, increased blood pressure and a higher risk of mental illness.

Stress cannot be entirely avoided so it is important to be able to recognise it when it becomes dangerous for health. It may be difficult to judge your own stress level on a day-to-day basis, however a cortisol test can provide a definite measurement to monitor. A home test kit typically involves taking a saliva swab several times over a day because cortisol levels should be highest just after waking and then fall throughout the day and are lowest at bedtime.

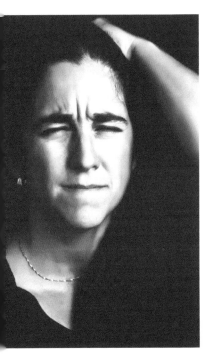

▷ Take control of situations that cause you stress

▷ Monitor your cortisol levels as an objective measure of stress

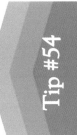

Tip #54

Information
10 stress busters
NHS - https://go22.uk/stressbusters

Stress Level Test
PSYCOM - https://go22.uk/psycom
3 Minute Test. NOTE: you don't have to enter your email address to get a result

Cortisol Tests
Lab Tests Online - https://go22.uk/cortisoltest

Perceived stress and cause-specific mortality among men and women
American Journal of Epidemiology - https://go22.uk/rp0571
Men with high stress versus low stress had higher all-cause mortality

Urinary Cortisol and Six-Year Risk of All-Cause and Cardiovascular Mortality
The Journal of Clinical Endocrinology & Metabolism - https://go22.uk/rp0572
High cortisol levels strongly predict cardiovascular death with and without pre-existing CVD

COST: ● ● ● ● ●   EASE: ● ● ● ○ ○   IMPACT: ● ● ● ○ ○

Volunteering

A great deal of research has been directed towards determining the effects of volunteering in older individuals. Results have been consistent in that field - to volunteer, to help others within the context of a greater cause, is considered a powerful tool for improving health in the elderly. Volunteering has been associated with lower mortality, better health and a lower incidence of depression.

Interestingly, not all forms of volunteering are the same. Those who have some kind of religious motivation tend to obtain greater benefits from the experience. Equally perplexing is the precise mechanism behind the beneficial effects of volunteering over the human body and how mental choices and lifestyle actions affect human biology.

Even though the "how" is not understood, volunteering is a simple and low-cost technique to increase healthspan, and there are a wide variety of causes, that are always looking for enthusiastic helpers.

Tip #55

▶ Volunteer for one or more organisations

▶ Try to do a volunteer activity at least once a week

▶ Pick a cause that will keep you motivated

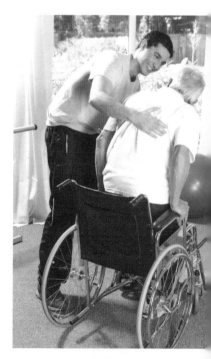

Information
The many ways volunteering is good for your heart
Harvard Health Blog - https://go22.uk/v4good

Organisations
Do-it - https://go22.uk/doit
Comprehensive list of volunteer opportunities with ability to search by location, cause (e.g. children, environment) and skills (e.g. interpersonal, IT, creative)

Volunteer abroad with VSO - https://go22.uk/vsoi

Volunteerism and Mortality among the Community-dwelling Elderly
Journal of Health Psychology - https://go22.uk/rp0961
High volunteers (>=2 organizations) had 44 percent lower mortality than non-volunteers

Caregiving, volunteering or both? Comparing effects on health and mortality
Age and Ageing - https://go22.uk/rp0962
Both caregiving and volunteering were separately associated with reduced mortality risk

COST: ● ● ● ○ ○   EASE: ● ● ● ○ ○   IMPACT: ● ● ○ ○ ○

Biological age

It is said that age is just a number, and this is so true, as chronological age does not determine how the body has aged. Scientific research has found that a person's chronological age does not correspond to the status of biological functions in their body.

The factor which determines the ageing of the body in the true sense is therefore its biological age. Studies show that biological age predicts mortality better than chronological age.

The parameters which are used to calculate biological age include behavioural, physical, and biomedical. The weight of the body, BMI, blood pressure, waist circumference, body fat percentage, body muscle percentage, frailty index, cholesterol levels, blood sugar, and urea nitrogen levels form the first line of ageing biomarkers which determine biological age.

Examining various attributes of an individual's DNA also enables scientists to determine biological age more accurately and hence to predict mortality. The telomeres' length, and modifications of the DNA (epigenetics) are among the many biomarkers, which reveal different aspects of the ageing process.

Not surprisingly, with so many factors, it can often be the case that different body parts age at different rates. For example, breast and lung tissue in females and skeletal muscle in males tend to be biologically older than the rest of the body.

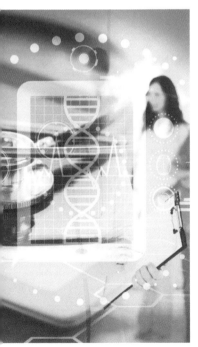

▷ Track your biological age with wide-ranging tests every few years
▷ Adjust your lifestyle based on your fastest ageing biomarkers

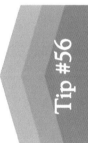

Tip #56

Information

Chronological v biological age infographic
Live Forever Club blog - https://go22.uk/biomarkers

What's your heart age? - https://go22.uk/heartage
NHS web test tells you your heart's biological age

Products

Deep Biomarkers Of Human Aging
Insilico Medicine - https://go22.uk/insilico
Enter blood test details to estimate biological age

myDNAge - https://go22.uk/mydnaage
Blood and urine tests to calculate biological age

The frailty index in Europeans: association with age and mortality
Age and Ageing - https://go22.uk/rp1071
Frailty Index (biological age parameter) predicts the mortality better than the chronological age

DNA methylation age of blood predicts all-cause mortality in later life
Genome Biology - https://go22.uk/rp1072
The status of DNA methylation predicts mortality better than chronological age

COST: ●●●●○   EASE: ●●●●○   IMPACT: ●●●○○

Blood pressure

Blood pressure (BP) is a vital sign that gives an estimation of the health of one's heart. A reading below 120/80 mmHg (systolic/diastolic pressure) is healthy, but one's target value varies by age, health, and medical history. Measurements above this correlate with various stages of high BP or hypertension. Values ranging between 140-159/90-99 mmHg denote hypertension stage 1 and requires attention towards remedies to control it.

One in four UK adults suffers from high blood pressure. Studies show that among individuals aged from 40 to 89, the risk of developing heart disease and stroke doubles with every 20mmHg and 10mmHg increase in systolic and diastolic pressure, respectively. High blood pressure elevates the risk of diabetes, kidney and eye damage, and has been associated with cognitive decline.

A range less than 90/60 mmHg is considered as a low BP and it comes with its own set of complications. The symptoms of low BP include dizziness, blurry vision, fainting and nausea or vomiting. It may be genetic or can be caused by anaemia, dehydration, pregnancy, and low blood sugar levels. Lower diastolic pressure has been associated with higher risk of dementia.

Blood pressure fluctuates throughout the day, but swings of more than 14 mm Hg between readings are associated with the severity of cardiovascular events, kidney damage, and all-cause mortality.

Tip #57

▶ Check your blood pressure every few months
▶ If high, make appropriate lifestyle changes to lower your blood pressure
▶ Readings above 180/120 should be treated as a medical emergency

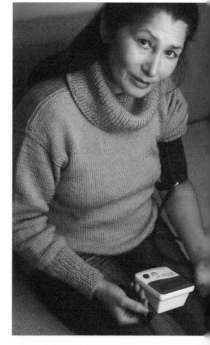

Information

Blood pressure chart
https://go22.uk/bpchart
Shows low, ideal and high ranges for both systolic and diastolic blood pressure.

Preventing High Blood Pressure - NHS
https://go22.uk/bpnhs

Products

Validated BP Monitors for Home Use – British and Irish Hypertension Society
https://go22.uk/bpmonitors

Relation of Blood Pressure and All-Cause Mortality in 180 000 Japanese Participants
Hypertension - https://go22.uk/rp0421
High blood pressure raised the risk of total mortality, higher in the younger population.

Lifestyle interventions to reduce raised blood pressure: a systematic review
Journal of Hypertension - https://go22.uk/rp0422
BP can be lowered by diet, exercise and restricting the use of alcohol and salt intake.

COST: ●● ○ ○ ○   EASE: ●●●● ○   IMPACT: ●●● ○ ○

Blood tests

Humans are currently faced with the consequences of having bodies susceptible to wearing out. The risk for chronic diseases, such as cancer, liver damage and heart disease tends to increase after the 40-year-old mark, but, regular testing can provide early warning of these conditions, providing time to tackle the problem before too much damage has been done.

Colon and breast cancer are complex conditions that tend to appear in older individuals, and in the case of colorectal cancer, this is especially true. Right now, there are a few blood tests that can be used for early diagnosis and monitoring. "Complete blood count" is useful for the detection of colon cancer. "Carcinoembryonic antigen (CEA)" blood levels are also useful for several different types of carcinomas including breast cancer.

Liver damage is also a frequent cause of death in the UK. Some of the most commonly used markers for acute or chronic liver damage are "AST and ALT" and most laboratories are able to measure them at a low cost.

The most useful markers for heart disease are "LDL, HDL and C-reactive protein" (usually evaluated together in the same test). Increased levels have been observed to have strong correlation with several cardiovascular conditions.

IUM
ASSIUM
LORIDE
RBON DIOXIDE
EA NITROGEN
REATININE
UN/CREATININE RATIO
RIC ACID
PHOSPHORUS
CALCIUM
CHOLESTEROL, TOTAL
HDL CHOLESTEROL
CHOLESTEROL/HDL RATIO
LDL CHOL, CALCULATED
See footnote 1
TRIGLYCERIDES

▶ Take a broad-ranging blood test every year or two

▶ Test more frequently for any results that are out of range

▶ Take action to bring out of range results back to normal

Tip #58

Information
Lab Tests Online - https://go22.uk/labtests
Non-commercial information on the background and procedure of most common tests.

Products
Medichecks - https://go22.uk/medichecks
Wide range of blood tests with a personal dashboard for reviewing and tracking results over time.

Thriva - https://go22.uk/thriva
Subscribe to regular testing with a simple at-home finger-prick blood test.

Circulating Oxidized LDL a Useful Marker for Identifying Patients With Coronary Artery Disease
Arteriosclerosis, Thrombosis, and Vascular Biology - https://go22.uk/rp0431
Circulating oxidized LDL is a sensitive marker of coronary artery disease

The value of a complete blood count in predicting cancer of the colon
Cancer Detection and Prevention - https://go22.uk/rp0432
An elevated red cell distribution width may help better identify referrals for full colonoscopy

COST: ● ● ○ ○ ○   EASE: ● ● ● ● ○   IMPACT: ● ● ○ ○ ○

DNA sequencing

DNA sequencing is the name given to reading small fragments of, or even the whole, DNA. Human DNA contains the code for around 20,000 genes that control how the body grows and operates. In terms of healthcare, the basis for personalised medicine lies in the information held in those genes. Commercially available gene testing kits can reveal whether an individual has a higher risk of certain diseases based on their genetic makeup.

Apart from some single gene disorders (e.g. cystic fibrosis, Huntington disease) the risk that a person will succumb to a disease does not solely depend on that person's genetic makeup, but also on their environment (such as income, education, relationships). Merely carrying a susceptibility gene does not necessarily imply one will develop the associated disease.

In cases of other fatal diseases such as cancer, coronary heart disease or diabetes, the environment plays a crucial role and hence prediction becomes more difficult. This is a new and evolving area, and as more data becomes available, the forecasting accuracy of DNA testing is likely to improve. However, for now the most accurate predictions come from combining DNA results with conventional risk factors.

Tip #59

▶ Take a DNA test – choose one that focuses on health, not ancestry

▶ If you are at higher risk of a condition then consider action to mitigate it

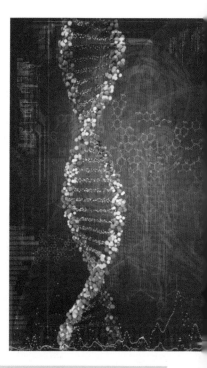

Information
Genetic Testing FAQ - https://go22.uk/geneticfaq
National Human Genome Research Institute

Genetic testing and counselling
NHS advice - https://go22.uk/geneticnhs

Products
23andMe – https://go22.uk/23andme
Health + Ancestry Service £149 (US$199)
Looks for 5 health risks, 40 carrier genes & 25 traits

Guide to Finding the Best DNA Health Test
Inner Body - https://go22.uk/dnahealth

Genetic Prediction of Future Type 2 Diabetes
PLoS Medicine - https://go22.uk/rp0441
Risk is more predictive when more genetic variants were taken into account

Candidate Gene Genotypes, Along with Conventional Risk Factor Assessment, Improve
Estimation of Coronary Heart Disease Risk in Healthy UK Men
Clinical Chemistry - https://go22.uk/rp0442

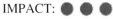

COST: ● ● ○ ○ ○   EASE: ● ● ● ○ ○   IMPACT: ● ● ● ○ ○

Health checks

The number of people diagnosed with chronic, noncommunicable diseases, such as atherosclerosis and cancer, are constantly on the rise, and the early detection of which usually leads to more cures or longer survival. To improve the chances of discovering problems early, many health bodies have come up with various health screening programmes for different age groups.

Currently, the NHS offers eight national screening programmes in England. As the saying goes, "prevention is better than cure," and studies have suggested that such health screening check-ups have resulted in a significant reduction in all-cause mortality rate.

Unfortunately, the NHS can only afford to offer the minimum possible screening, for example the general "Health Check" is only available to those aged 40-74 every five years. It's designed to spot early signs of stroke, kidney disease, heart disease, type 2 diabetes or dementia – all of which would be better to find sooner rather than later.

Private health checks can also offer a wider range of tests, with your budget the only limit – Human Longevity's Health Nucleus test comes in at $25,000 and includes a complete genome sequence, a full-body MRI scan, a cardio CT scan, and more. But there are plenty of companies offering affordable health check-ups that include assessments which are difficult to perform yourself at home, such as ECG, musculoskeletal and lung function tests.

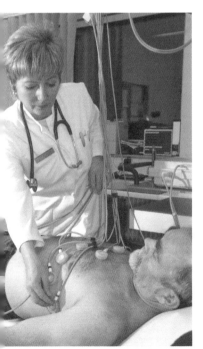

▷ Get a health check that suits your budget every couple of years

▷ If you already have symptoms, visit a doctor

▷ Track the results to spot unexpected changes

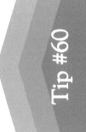

Tip #60

Information

Thinking of having a private screening test?
NHS leaflet - https://go22.uk/screening

Products

Bupa health assessments –
https://go22.uk/bupaassess
From £184 (~US$235). All health assessments include two follow-up calls with a health coach

Nuffield health assessments –
https://go22.uk/nuffield
From £267 (~US$340). Results given straight away, with time to review them during your assessment

NHS health checks through general practice: randomised trial of cardiovascular risk reduction
BMC Public Health - https://go22.uk/rp1121
Health check-ups significantly reduce the risk of cardiovascular disease

Preventive health screenings and health consultations in primary care increase life expectancy without increasing costs
Scandinavian Journal of Public Health - https://go22.uk/rp1122

COST: EASE: ● ● ● ● ○   IMPACT:

Telomeres

Inside the body's cells, DNA is condensed into twenty-three pairs of chromosomes during cell division. The tip of each chromosome is a telomere, a region of repeated DNA that marks the ends. Telomeres protect the chromosomes from deterioration and maintain their genomic structure, in the same way as plastic tips prevent the ends of shoelaces from fraying.

Unfortunately, telomeres shorten every time cells divide. When the telomere is too short, cells can no longer divide, and ageing accelerates. Lifestyle factors such as smoking, alcohol consumption, sleeping quality, exercise, and stress can greatly influence the shortening rate of the telomere.

Telomere length is therefore a good way to measure biological age. The shorter the telomeres, the higher the risk factor of some diseases such as cardiovascular diseases, Alzheimer's, diabetes, and cancer. Tracking telomere lengths can help determine whether lifestyle interventions are being effective, and help predict someone's life expectancy. This may sway how much effort is put into one's life extension plan of attack.

STOP PRESS: breaking research hints that it may be that the shape of telomeres is more important than their length.

Tip #61

▶ Have your telomeres tested every few years to track your biological age
▶ If telomeres are short, or decreasing rapidly, then make lifestyle changes
▶ Consider telomere lengthening therapies

Information
Are Telomeres the Key to Aging and Cancer?
University of Utah - https://go22.uk/utahtelo

Products
Accu-metrics Telomere Test - £79
Cheek swab test - https://go22.uk/viamedex1

TeloYears Telomere Health DNA Test – US$99
Finger blood drop test - https://go22.uk/teloyears

Telomerase & Myostatin Inhibition treatement
Provided by IHS in partnership with BioViva -
https://go22.uk/bioviva1

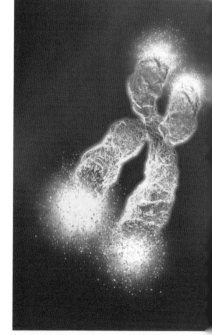

Peripheral blood leukocyte telomere length and mortality among 64,637 individuals
JNCI: Journal of the National Cancer Institute - https://go22.uk/rp0451
Short telomeres are associated with all-cause mortality

Short Telomere Length and Ischemic Heart Disease: Observational and Genetic Studies
Clinical Chemistry - https://go22.uk/rp0452
Short telomeres are associated with a higher risk of ischemic heart disease

COST: ● ● ● ● ●   EASE: ● ● ● ● ●   IMPACT: ● ● ● ○ ○

Visual checks

The earlier a disease is discovered, the easier it is to treat. Skin cancers, for example, found and removed early are almost always curable. Sometimes symptoms are few and hard to spot, so it is important to make an extra effort to look for early signs.

Studies have shown that self-examination is key to improving chances of survival and is associated with reduced mortality. Regular visual checks of the body can reveal precancerous lesions of breast cancer, testicular cancer, oral cancer and skin cancer. Therefore, the Skin Cancer Foundation recommends that everyone practices monthly head-to-toe self-examinations to find any new or changing lesions.

The visual checks in breast self-examination should focus on any change in the size or shape of the breast, a new lump, bleeding from the nipple, or a rash on or around the nipple that does not heal quickly.

For testicular self-examination, one should look for the formation of a lump in the testicle, any swelling in the testicle, a dull ache in the groin, or any deposition of fluid in the scrotum.

ABCDE rule for the early detection of melanoma

Asymmetry

Borders
(the outer edges are uneven)

Color
(dark black or have multiple colors)

Diameter
(greater than 6 mm)
(6 mm)

Evolving
(change in size, shape and color)

▷ Examine your body every three months
▷ Check your breasts or testicles for lumps
▷ Check your skin and mouth for lesions
▷ If you find any indication of a disease, visit a doctor as soon as possible

Tip #62

Information

How should I check my breasts?
NHS - https://go22.uk/nhsbreasts

What should my testicles look and feel like?
NHS - https://go22.uk/nhstesticles

Step by Step Self-Examination
Skin Cancer Foundation - https://go22.uk/skinexam

Intra Oral Self-Exam
Six step screening - https://go22.uk/oralexam

Breast self-examination and death from breast cancer: a meta-analysis
British Journal of Cancer - https://go22.uk/rp0461
Regular Breast Self Examination (BSE) leads to early detection and reduced mortality

Sun Exposure and Mortality From Melanoma
Journal of the National Cancer Institute - https://go22.uk/rp0462
Individuals who reported skin awareness were at significantly lower risk of death from melanoma

COST: ● ● ● ● ○   EASE: ● ● ● ● ●   IMPACT: ● ● ● ○ ○

Weight

Maintaining a healthy weight is one of the fundamental approaches to longevity and lowering the risks of serious diseases. Although the more common problem is being overweight, being underweight is also associated with a higher risk of infectious disease, cognitive issues, premature death and pregnancy problems.

In the UK, 41% of adults are overweight or obese (while 2% are underweight) and that figure is 57% in the US. Being overweight can lead to a long list of health risks including diabetes, cardiometabolic conditions, stroke, cancers, respiratory conditions and reduced quality of life. Many of these conditions lead to a premature death with an estimated 30,000 deaths annually in the UK associated with obesity.

Although the body mass index (BMI) is widely-used to categorise people's weight, recent research has found that the waist-hip ratio (WHR) is a more relevant measure of actual body fat levels. WHR also turns out to be more accurate than BMI for predicting health risks, possibly because belly fat is the real criminal in risks associated with obesity.

All weight loss diets, however they are dressed up, work on the principle of burning more calories than are consumed – however, given the number of overweight people it is obviously not simple to put into practice. The mental strength needed to adhere to a diet should not be underestimated.

Tip #63

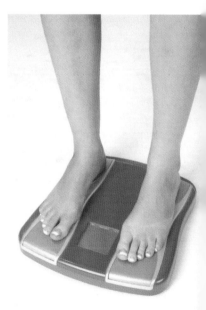

▶ Weigh yourself weekly – ideally with scales that also measure fat percentage

▶ Measure your waist to hip ratio monthly

▶ Aim for a waist to hip ratio of under 0.85 (women) or 0.9 (men)

Information
Obesity - https://go22.uk/nhsobesity
NHS advice including causes, diagnosis and treatment for obesity

What Is the Waist-to-Hip Ratio? How to measure it
Healthline - https://go22.uk/waisthip

Products
Waist to Hip Ratio Calculator
https://go22.uk/whrcalc

10 Best Body Fat Scales Tested And Fully Reviewed
Runner Click - https://go22.uk/10fatscales

Body mass index, waist circumference and waist-hip ratio: which is the better discriminator of cardiovascular disease mortality risk?
Obesity Reviews - https://go22.uk/rp0471
Measures of WHR, but not BMI, were related to an increased risk of CVD mortality

COST: ● ● ● ● ●   EASE: ● ● ● ● ●   IMPACT: ● ● ○ ○ ○

Aspirin

Many research studies have concluded that aspirin can help with cancer prevention (especially in the case of lung and colorectal cancer) and it is beneficial in the prevention of cardiovascular disease.

It is important to realise that aspirin provides this kind of protection only in the long-term, meaning that an individual must incorporate aspirin in his/her routine over a period of time for it to take effect. It is believed that the preventive effects start after at least five years of continuous supplementation.

However, one must be careful. Because aspirin is a blood thinner, taking large doses of it for long periods of time can cause mild or even severe bleeding in the elderly and those prone to haemorrhage. The dose that provides the optimal balance of benefits and risk is still to be agreed in the scientific community.

Under conditions of prolonged low-dose consumption, the risk of cancer can be reduced up to 40%. The best results have been achieved with a daily consumption of about 100 mg of aspirin tablets with an enteric coating (which allows them to pass through the stomach to the small intestine before dissolving) for an average of ten years.

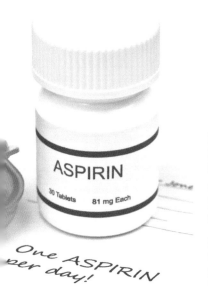

▶ Talk with your doctor about whether long-term low-dose aspirin consumption might be suitable for you
▶ The benefits may only outweigh the harm if you have a higher risk of heart disease

Tip #64

Information
Daily aspirin therapy: benefits and risks
Mayo Clinic - https://go22.uk/dailyasp

Low dose aspirin - https://go22.uk/lowasp
NHS information including cautions with other medicines

Products
What Smart People Never Buy At The Drugstore
Huffington Post - https://go22.uk/genericasp
Typical shoppers choose pricier brand-name aspirin, even though it's essentially the same

Low-Dose Aspirin or Nonsteroidal Anti-inflammatory Drug Use and Colorectal Cancer Risk
Annals of Internal Medicine - https://go22.uk/rp0111
Long-term use of low-dose aspirin and NSAIDs associated with reduced colorectal cancer risk

Which Aspirin Dose and Preparation is Best for the Long-Term Prevention of CVD and Cancer?
Progress in Cardiovascular Diseases - https://go22.uk/rp0112
Daily dose of 100 mg of coated aspirin confer favourable preventive effects on death and cancer

COST: ● ● ● ● ○   EASE: ● ● ● ● ●   IMPACT: ● ● ● ○ ○

Coenzyme Q10

Coenzyme Q10 (CoQ10) is a natural antioxidant synthesised in the body's cells. It's essential for energy production, longevity and healthy ageing, but its levels diminish as people age. Small quantities of CoQ10 are available in meat, fish and wholegrains but it is not possible to significantly increase CoQ10 levels in the body from dietary sources.

As low Coenzyme Q10 levels have been associated with heart disease, it may be necessary to supplement the body's reserves. As the body does not store CoQ10 it needs to be part of a daily regime.

CoQ10 supplementation is able to support the heart by improving blood flow and helping to maintain blood pressure within a healthy range. In addition, its anti-inflammatory properties lower the risk of heart problems associated with chronic inflammation. In addition, CoQ10 protects the heart from the negative effects of chemotherapy drugs and statin medications.

Coenzyme Q10 may play a role in reducing the symptoms of Parkinson's disease and Alzheimer's with no known side-effects.

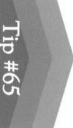

Tip #65

▶ Take 100 milligrams of Coenzyme Q10 daily (or less in ubiquinol form)

▶ Include a form of fat in your meal because CoQ10 is fat soluble

▶ Speak to your doctor if you are taking anticoagulants (blood-thinning drugs)

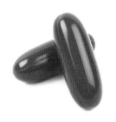

Information
9 Benefits of Coenzyme Q10 (CoQ10) - Healthline
https://go22.uk/coq10

What is the difference between CoQ10 and ubiquinol? - Consumer Lab
https://go22.uk/ubiquinol

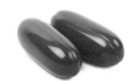

Products
Best CoQ10 Supplement (Reviews & Buyers Guide)
BiohackersLab - https://go22.uk/coq10review

100mg Coenzyme Q10 – from 15p each (US$0.20)
Just Vitamins - https://go22.uk/coq10capsules

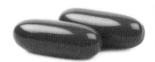

Reduced Cardiovascular Mortality 10 Years after Supplementation with Selenium and Coenzyme Q10 for Four Years
PLOS ONE - https://go22.uk/rp0281

Effects of coenzyme Q10 supplementation on inflammatory markers: A systematic review
Pharmacological Research - https://go22.uk/rp0282
Coenzyme Q10 supplementation significantly lowers inflammatory markers in blood

COST: ●●●○○   EASE: ●●●●●   IMPACT: ●●○○○

Lithium

Lithium is recommended as a treatment for several mental health disorders because of its mood-stabilising properties. However, this particular element has other hidden properties and characteristics that could be useful.

Firstly, lithium is not a molecule or compound, it's an element (a metal) in the periodic table and its most common form is known as Li+, an ion usually found at very low concentration in some sources of water. Although, typically around 100 litres would need to be drunk to consume the same amount of lithium prescribed for medical purposes.

Low dose lithium consumption has been shown to provide a protective effect for human health and life extension. This is based on studies that have compared average lifespan in populations with different lithium levels in their drinking water. People in communities whose water has a concentration of around 0.4 mg/l of lithium chloride (LiCl) tend to live longer.

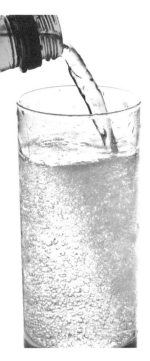

▷ Aim for around 1 milligram of lithium per day
▷ Test your home drinking water for lithium content – it may be sufficient
▷ Increase your intake by drinking mineral water or taking supplements

Tip #66

Information
Mark My Words, There Will Be An RDA For Lithium In The Future
Fanatic Cook - https://go22.uk/lithium

Products
Gerolsteiner mineral water -
https://go22.uk/gerolsteiner
Lithium: 0.13 mg/litre

San Pelligrino mineral water -
https://go22.uk/pelligrino
Lithium: 0.12 mg/litre

Low-dose lithium uptake promotes longevity in humans and metazoans
European Journal of Nutrition - https://go22.uk/rp0621
Low-dose exposure to lithium decreases mortality in evolutionary distinct species

Lithium: occurrence, dietary intakes, nutritional essentiality
Journal of the American College of Nutrition - https://go22.uk/rp0622
Evidence appears to accept lithium as essential; provisional RDA for a 70 kg adult of 1 mg/day

COST: ● ● ● ○ ○   EASE: ● ● ● ● ●   IMPACT: ● ● ● ○ ○

Nicotinamide riboside (NR)

Nicotinamide riboside (NR) is one of the three forms of vitamin B3 and a biological precursor that, through a couple of reactions, transforms into NAD+ which is a vital coenzyme found in all living cells. Nicotinamide adenine dinucleotide (NAD) enables many reactions within the cells and particularly aids the function of power-generating mitochondria.

However, levels of the oxidised form of NAD (NAD+) decrease in cells with age, contributing to many age-associated diseases. So, researchers have investigated the effect of boosting NAD+ levels – and, at least in mice, this has rejuvenated cells resulting in improved insulin production and regulation, decreased retinal degeneration and the reversal of vascular ageing.

As well as being created in the body, NAD+ can be synthesised in various ways from the intake of food.Studies have shown that consumption of NR results in an increased level of NAD+ in multiple tissues.

Another precursor is nicotinamide mononucleotide (NMN), which has seen similarly successful results in mice and that is currently in a small-scale human trial run by David Sinclair of Harvard Medical School.

Tip #67

▶ Consider including NR as part of your daily supplement regime
▶ Safe levels are yet to be determined, so for now limit to 300 mg/day

Information
Do NAD-Boosting Supplements Fight Aging?
Berkeley Wellness - https://go22.uk/nadboosting

Results from a Preliminary Human Trial of Nicotinamide Riboside Supplementation
Fighting Aging! - https://go22.uk/nrsupps

Products
Best Nicotinamide Riboside Supplement (Reviews & Buyers Guide)
Biohackers Lab - https://go22.uk/nrguide

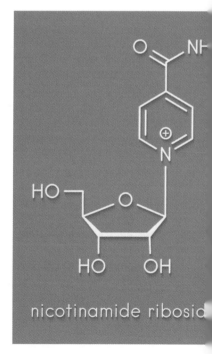

nicotinamide ribosid

Age-Associated Changes In Oxidative Stress and NAD+ Metabolism In Human Tissue
PLoS One - https://go22.uk/rp0041
NAD+ depletion may limit energy production, DNA repair and genomic signalling

Nicotinamide riboside is uniquely and orally bioavailable in mice and humans
Nature Communications - https://go22.uk/rp0042
Supplementation enables clinical translation of NR to improve wellness & treat human diseases

COST: ●●●●○ EASE: ●●●●● IMPACT: ●●●●○

Phosphatidylcholine

Phosphatidylcholine (PC) is an important structural component of cellular membranes in the body – composing about 90% of the membrane in children. However, because the body makes it very slowly, this drops to only 10% in the elderly.

PC, like all fatty components of cell membranes, suffer damage over time and need to be replaced, but this mechanism loses its effectiveness with age. Reduced PC can lead to several disorders in the brain and liver.

Phosphatidylcholine is found in foods, including eggs, sunflowers, soy, and mustard, and can also be taken as a supplement. When ingested with other nutrients it increases their bioavailability, making them more effective too.

It has been found that PC can lead to an improvement in some key aspects of memory, learning, ageing and fatigue. In the last few years, supplementing PC has been discussed as an important component in treatments against brain pathologies such as Alzheimer's and Parkinson's disease.

In Ray Kurzweil's book, Transcend ("nine steps to living well forever"), he recommends that everyone starts taking this supplement immediately to slow down ageing, so it should be considered seriously.

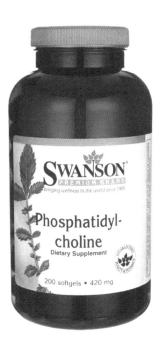

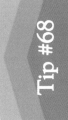

▷ Include phosphatidylcholine as part of your daily supplement regime
▷ Daily values are not yet determined, so for now limit to 2,000 mg/day
▷ Phosphatidylcholine may be particularly beneficial to vegans

Tip #68

Information
Uses, side effects, interactions & dosing information
WebMD - https://go22.uk/phosphat1

Get Smarter: A Powerful Brain-Boosting Supplement You've Never Heard Of
Forbes - https://go22.uk/phosphat2

Products
Supplements - 420 mg, 90 softgels - £14 (US$20)
Natural Factors - https://go22.uk/phosphatnf

Supplements - 420 mg, 200 softgels - £23 (US$25)
Swanson Premium - https://go22.uk/phosphatsp

Pilot Study: Reduction of Fatigue by Use of a Dietary Supplement Containing Glycophospholipids
Journal of the American Nutraceutical Association - https://go22.uk/rp0021
Dietary supplementation of phosphatidylcholine significantly reduced fatigue

COST: ●●●● ○   EASE: ●●●●●   IMPACT: ●● ○ ○ ○

Resveratrol

Resveratrol is a chemical compound found in red wine, and is also present in cranberries, raspberries, peanuts and blackberries. Some of the benefits associated with resveratrol have been anti-inflammatory effects, immune-modulation, and anti-carcinogenic properties. There has been considerable debate and research regarding this molecule, sufficient to prompt large pharmaceutical companies to initiate human trials to determine its health benefits.

Resveratrol has a complex behaviour in different organisms, which means any research results with non-human models does not necessarily apply to humans. In fact, it has been revealed that most experiments and trials that reported beneficial results in animals, used high doses of resveratrol that are dangerous to humans, since they can cause renal problems. The ideal dose and the best means of consumption are still not clear.

There is something both positive and interesting to be said about the ingestion of resveratrol through wine. Light drinkers of red wine tend to have lower occurrence of coronary heart disease, which aligns with a low ingestion of resveratrol. Some scientists believe it is behind the "French paradox" whereby French people have a low incidence of heart disease despite eating comparatively rich diets.

Tip #69

▶ Consider including 30 mg of resveratrol as part of your daily supplement regime
▶ If you choose to drink alcohol, make it a small glass of red wine to get a resveratrol bonus

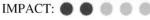

Information
7 Health Benefits of Resveratrol Supplements
Healthline - https://go22.uk/resver7

Red wine and resveratrol: Good for your heart?
Mayo Clinic - https://go22.uk/redwine

Products
Supplements on Amazon – from £2.66 (~$3.50) for 50mg, 30 Capsules - https://go22.uk/resversup

Resveratrol Powder
Bulk Powders - https://go22.uk/resverbp
Claims to be highest purity at 99% trans-resveratrol

resveratrol

Resveratrol supplementation improves glycemic control in type 2 diabetes mellitus
Nutrition Research - https://go22.uk/rp0591
Oral supplementation of Resveratrol is thus found to be effective in improving glycemic control

Mechanism of cardioprotection by Resveratrol, a phenolic antioxidant present in red wine
International Journal of Molecular Medicine - https://go22.uk/rp0592
Light consumption can reduce severity of atherosclerosis and risk for coronary heart disease

COST: ● ● ● ● ○   EASE: ● ● ● ● ●   IMPACT: ● ● ○ ○ ○

Turmeric (curcumin)

Curcumin is the most active substance in turmeric, the main spice in curry. With more than 10,000 scientific studies, curcumin has been demonstrated to be an effective supplement to control disorders of ageing.

Curcumin is among the most potent anti-inflammatory compounds and can help control chronic inflammation that leads to serious diseases such as cancer, cardiovascular, and neurodegenerative diseases. It does this by blocking key signalling molecules (NF-kB) in the inflammatory pathway.

Another mechanism behind ageing are oxidative agents which damage DNA and destroy cells. Curcumin has a powerful antioxidant action (neutralises free radicals) in that it inhibits lipid oxidation in cell membranes.

With its anti-inflammatory and antioxidant activities, curcumin acts as a neuroprotective agent - helping to protect from common neurodegenerative diseases associated with ageing such as Alzheimer's and Parkinson's disease. It also increases the level of BDNF, a hormone that enhances the neuron activity.

Curcumin also helps lower the risk of cardiovascular diseases. It improves the function of the vascular endothelium (cells that line blood vessels) thereby helping to prevent the development of atherosclerosis and other arterial diseases.

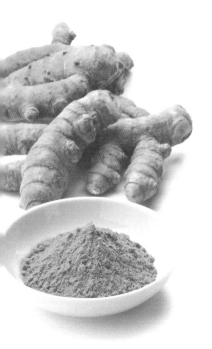

▷ Use turmeric in your cooking – it's mild so blends in with most flavours
▷ Consuming with fats may boost the absorption of its curcumin
▷ Take a 1,000 mg supplement on days turmeric is missing from your diet

Tip #70

Information
Could turmeric really boost your health?
BBC - https://go22.uk/turmeric

Turmeric vs Curcumin: Which Should You Take?
Healthline - https://go22.uk/curcumin

Products
Nature's Garden Turmeric 400mg 100 Capsules - £15.99 (~US$21)
Holland and Barrett - https://go22.uk/hbturmeric
They are regularly on offer so wait for a 2-for-1 or shop around

Phase IIA Clinical Trial of Curcumin for the Prevention of Colorectal Neoplasia
Cancer Prevention Research - https://go22.uk/rp0291
Curcumin extracts able to suppress carcinogenesis, could be used as a cancer prevention agent

Efficacy of Turmeric Extracts and Curcumin for Alleviating the Symptoms of Joint Arthritis
Journal of Medicinal Food - https://go22.uk/rp0292
Curcumin extract is significantly effective for arthritis pain and reduced need for medication

COST: ● ● ● ● ●   EASE: ● ● ● ● ●   IMPACT: ● ● ● ● ○

Vitamin D

Vitamin D is commonly linked to strong bones and muscles. However, studies have shown that its benefits extend to other health benefits, and that its intake also lowers overall mortality.

The protective role of vitamin D spreads over the entire life span. From early childhood to old age, sufficient intake of vitamin D prevents the occurrence of rickets, and reduces the risk of viral and bacterial infections, respiratory infections, cardiovascular diseases, inflammation and dementia. One study found a 77% reduction in cancer in those consuming the right levels of vitamin D and calcium.

Few foods are naturally rich in vitamin D, with the main source of vitamin D being its synthesis in the skin from sunlight. However, in the UK sunlight-induced vitamin D synthesis is only effective between April and September but not throughout the winter months. Supplementation is therefore recommended for anyone living above or below 37 degrees latitude – roughly San Francisco-Athens-Beijing in the northern hemisphere and Buenos Aires-Melbourne-Auckland in the south.

A concentration of vitamin D in serum (the part of the blood that contains no clotting factors or blood cells) below 25 nanomoles per litre (nm/L) depicts poor musculoskeletal health, with the normal range being between 50-200 nm/L.

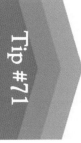

Tip #71

▶ Take a 10 microgram vitamin D supplement each day
▶ Don't take more than 100 micrograms per day as it could be harmful
▶ Monitor the vitamin D level in your blood using the 25(OH)D test

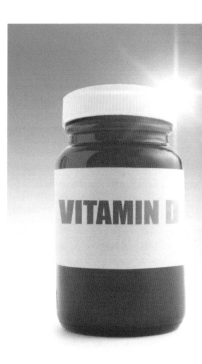

Information
Vitamin D and Health - https://go22.uk/vitdhealth
Harvard T.H. Chan School of Public Health

NHS information on sources, supplements, deficiency and taking too much vitamin D - https://go22.uk/vitdnhs

Products
Best Vitamin D Supplements
Consumer Reports - https://go22.uk/vitdsupps

Vitamin D 10 µg 90 tablets - £2.29 (~US$3)
Boots - https://go22.uk/vitdboots

Vitamin D and risk of cause specific death: systematic review and meta-analysis
BMJ - https://go22.uk/rp0051
Lower intake of vitamin D supplements led to higher risk of mortality

Vitamin D and calcium supplementation reduces cancer risk: results of a randomized trial
The American Journal of Clinical Nutrition - https://go22.uk/rp0052
Improving calcium and vitamin D nutritional status substantially reduces all-cancer risk

COST: ● ● ● ● ●   EASE: ● ● ● ● ●   IMPACT: ● ● ○ ○ ○

Vitamin E

Free radical production is an unwanted biproduct of the body's metabolism. Human cells have a built-in antioxidant system that prevents mutations and tissue damage during most of our lives, however, as with many things, it loses its effectiveness with age and oxidative damage becomes more noticeable. Vitamin E is part of the body's natural antioxidant system and hence supplementation can be particularly beneficial to the elderly and can also reduce cognitive decline.

Vitamin E provides protection against free radicals in general, but its main function is against the production of oxidised LDL (bad cholesterol). Decreased levels are associated with an increased risk of cardiovascular disease, hyperlipidemia and oxidative damage. It can also lead to more severe symptoms of ageing, lower sperm motility and reduced protection against the sun's UV rays.

Vitamin E is actually a group of eight related compounds - four tocopherols and four tocotrienols. Supplements that only contain alpha-tocopherol can actually have a negative impact on a more important vitamin E type called gamma-tocopherol. Therefore it is important to choose a supplement that includes all four tocopherols (alpha, beta, gamma, delta) and ideally all four tocotrienols too.

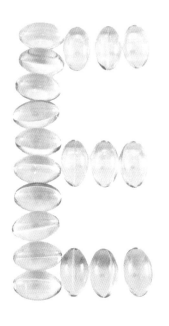

▷ Take a 50mg (75 IU) multi-component vitamin E supplement daily

▷ Include foods rich in vitamin E in your diet such as sunflower seeds, avocado and mango

Tip #72

Information
Vitamin E – NHS information - https://go22.uk/vitenhs
Taking 540mg or less a day of vitamin E supplements is unlikely to cause any harm

Products
Road Test: Vitamin E Supplements
Howl at the Moon - https://go22.uk/vitesupps
Great list of branded supplements including their gamma-tocopherol content

Meta-Analysis: High-Dosage Vitamin E Supplementation May Increase All-Cause Mortality
Annals of Internal Medicine - https://go22.uk/rp0631
For dosages less than 150 IU/d, all-cause mortality slightly but nonsignificantly decreased

Vitamin E and Cognitive Decline in Older Persons
Archives of Neurology - https://go22.uk/rp0632
Vitamin E intake, from foods or supplements, is associated with less cognitive decline with age

COST: ● ● ○ ○ ○   EASE: ● ● ● ○ ○   IMPACT: ● ● ○ ○ ○

Natural disasters

The chances of dying in a natural disaster are very low, but they can be reduced with a few precautions. Firstly, avoid living in areas of high risk – for example, California is due a big earthquake which could result in thousands of deaths. Secondly, if disaster does strike, here are the recommended actions to improve your chances of survival.

Avalanche - Shelter behind rocks or trees. Attempt to swim through the snow. Before impact, take in a deep breath and cover your nose and mouth. Use your arms to make an air space in front of your face. **Earthquake** – Drop (to your knees), cover (e.g. under a strong desk, or next to an interior wall) and hold (onto your shelter). If you are outside, move away from buildings, trees, and power lines. **Flooding** – Avoid narrow gullies which can flood many miles away from the rain storm. Don't drive or walk through moving flood waters. **Hurricane** – Evacuate if told to do so. Bring anything loose inside. Secure doors, windows and shutters. Stay away from windows. A lull may be the storm's eye - not its end. **Tornado** – Use TV, radio and apps to stay informed. Find shelter. Crouch low, face downward. Use blankets, mattresses, etc, to protect yourself from flying debris. **Tsunami** – Move to higher ground. If you are in the water, then grab onto something that floats. The largest surge may occur hours after the first wave. **Volcano** - Avoid areas downstream of the eruption. Seek shelter indoors if possible. Hold a damp cloth over your face. Wear goggles or glasses, not contact lenses. Avoid driving in heavy ash fall.

Tip #73

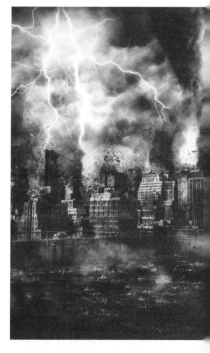

▸ Practice an evacuation plan with everyone in your family

▸ Stay alert – spot natural signs and listen for official warnings

▸ Maintain a disaster survival kit to last 3 days without power, water or food

Information

Cities Most Likely to Be Hit by An Earthquake
World Atlas - https://go22.uk/earthcities

Plan Ahead for Disasters - Department of Homeland Security - https://go22.uk/planahead

Products

The Natural Disaster Survival Handbook
Amazon - https://go22.uk/ndsurvival

Earthquake & Natural Disaster Survival Kit
EVAQ8 - https://go22.uk/evaq8kit

Survival Capsule - https://go22.uk/capsule

Immediate behavioural responses to earthquakes in Christchurch, NZ, and Hitachi, Japan
Disasters - https://go22.uk/rp0401
The most frequent response of residents in both cities was to freeze

Factors affecting survival in tsunami evacuation
Cambridge Architectural Research - https://go22.uk/rp0402
After 2011 earthquake many people went home, often into danger

COST: ● ● ● ○ ○   EASE: ● ● ● ○ ○   IMPACT: ● ● ● ○ ○

Pandemics

Throughout its history the world has faced the wrath of pandemics such as Spanish Flu, H1N1 Swine Flu, SARS, Ebola, and H5N1 Bird Flu, which have claimed millions of lives. These are highly unpredictable in their occurrence and their associated symptoms owing to their biological novelty. Pandemics are caused by novel virus strains, which are easily transmissible and against which humans have little or no immunity.

Flu pandemics generally display a variety of symptoms such as eye infections, pneumonia, vomiting, diarrhoea, severe respiratory diseases, and multi-organ failure, which often become the primary cause of death. Fatality rates during a pandemic can be appallingly high, with 50% of people infected with Ebola dying and even higher for bird flu. The number of deaths is often higher in older, weaker, individuals – although the overall fatality rate for SARS was 15% this jumped to 50% in persons aged 65 years and older.

To prevent social and economic disruption, the UK's pandemic response strategy is to make antiviral drugs available to people who have been in contact with an infected person. In the very early stages of a pandemic this is expected to reduce hospitalisations and save lives. However, there are actions an individual can take to reduce their chances of infection as well as to reduce the spread amongst the community.

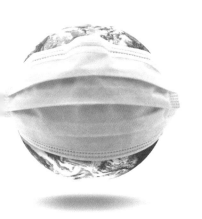

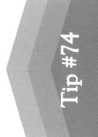

▶ Stockpile antiviral medications in case of shortage

▶ Prepare emergency kit (mask, gloves, disinfectant) if pandemic imminent

▶ During a pandemic avoid sick people and wash your hands often

Tip #74

Information

'Disease X': the mystery malady that could one day kill millions
Newsweek - https://go22.uk/diseasex

HealthMap - https://go22.uk/healthmap
Real-time intelligence on a broad range of emerging infectious diseases

How to Prepare for Pandemic
Happy Preppers - https://go22.uk/how2pandemic

How to avoid catching a virus on a plane
Science Mag - https://go22.uk/virusplane

Containing Pandemic Influenza with Antiviral Agents
American Journal of Epidemiology - https://go22.uk/rp0381
Has potential as an effective measure for containing influenza until vaccine is available

Nonpharmaceutical Interventions for Pandemic Influenza, National and Community Measures
Emerging Infectious Diseases - https://go22.uk/rp0382
Contaminated household surfaces should be disinfected

COST: ●● ● ● ●   EASE: ●● ● ● ●   IMPACT: ●● ● ● ●

Prepping

Whereas natural disaster preparation (see previous tip) is all about surviving a short-term catastrophe, prepping is about getting ready for the apocalypse – the total destruction of society. In practice, this means being prepared for at least two weeks without help, rather than just seventy-two hours. It took over a week for everyone to be reached after Hurricane Katrina.

The scenarios that preppers are making provisions for, are events that would cause society as we know it to break down, and therefore government and other agencies cannot be relied upon to come to your aid. This level of devastation could be caused by an exceptional natural disaster (for example, a meteor impact or a super-volcano eruption), artificial intelligence take-over, ecological collapse, nuclear war or financial meltdown.

This may sound implausible to some, but with today's supply chains stripped down to bare efficiencies, it would not take long for chaos to break out. In 2000, a few hundred protesters blocked several key oil facilities in the UK; within a week, supermarkets were rationing bread, hospitals were cancelling operations and the army was called in to help.

The tools you'd need to stay alive will vary on where you live. Survival skills, such as hunting and gathering will be essential in rural areas. But for the 80% of the population that live in urban areas, scavenging, weapons, and negotiating will be far more useful.

Tip #75

▶ Be prepared for two weeks of societal breakdown

▶ Don't tell everyone about your preparations – you won't have enough to share

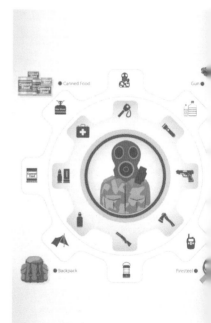

Canned Food   Gun   Backpack   Firesteel

Information
Emergency Preparedness Checklist for Beginners
The Prepared - https://go22.uk/preplist

Organisations
Global Catastrophic Risk Institute – analyses risks to the survival of human civilisation - https://go22.uk/gcri

Products
The Knowledge – How to rebuild our world from scratch - Lewis Dartnell
Amazon - https://go22.uk/knowledge

Human and nature dynamics: Modeling inequality and resources in the collapse of societies
Ecological Economics - https://go22.uk/rp0391
The new dynamics of this model can also reproduce the irreversible collapses found in history

Complexity and the productivity of innovation
Behavioral Science - https://go22.uk/rp0392
The results suggest that the conventional optimistic view may be unwarranted

COST: ● ● ● ● ●   EASE: ● ● ● ○ ○   IMPACT: ● ● ○ ○ ○

Self defence

The best form of self-defence is not putting yourself in a position where you have to defend yourself. Keep in mind that, according to statistics from England and Wales, in 60% of homicides the principal suspect was known to the victim. Half of all female victims were killed by partners or ex-partners, with less than one in ten being killed by a total stranger. Many of these deaths were the result of a quarrel or a revenge attack.

In the UK, where gun ownership is restricted, knife usage, strangulation and kicking are the most common methods of killing.

While out in public areas, always be aware of your surroundings and the people around you. If attacked try to run from the attacker. If it's not possible to get away, then shout for attention and use your personal alarm if you have one. Ultimately, and if handing over your valuables has not appeased your assailant, then attack them with maximum force directed at their weak body points (i.e. eyes, nose, throat, groin, knees), hopefully giving you a chance to get away.

NOTE: pepper spray is illegal in the UK (and regarded as a firearm), however its sale is unrestricted in some other European countries.

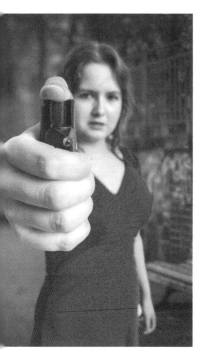

▶ Buy a personal attack alarm and a legal self-defence spray
▶ Learn some basic self-defence techniques
▶ Avoid dangerous places and people

Tip #76

Information
Avoidance, Awareness, & Prevention
David Erath Jr - https://go22.uk/avoidance
Learn how to stop assaults before they begin

Basic Self-Defense Moves Anyone Can Do
Life Hacker - https://go22.uk/basicmoves

Products
REPELL Attack Deterrent Foul Dye - from £6 (US$8)
Walk Easy - https://go22.uk/walkeasy

Personal Alarms from £6 (US$8)
Suzy Lamplugh Trust - https://go22.uk/persalarms

Homicide in England and Wales: year ending March 2017
Office for National Statistics - https://go22.uk/rp0971
22% of adult male victims were killed by strangers, compared with 9% of female victims

COST: ●●●●● EASE: ●●●●● IMPACT: ●● ● ● ●

Air travel

The fastest and safest way to travel is flying. Though many people fear air crashes, statistics from UK Department for Transport show that there have been zero fatalities in commercial air transport since 2015, whereas there are around 1,700 road deaths every year.

Still, aircraft accidents do happen, and everyone should be prepared to increase their survival chances. Keep in mind that the European Transport Safety Council states that 90% of air accidents are survivable or technically survivable.

One fifth of air casualties are due to impact and another one fifth die because of smoke, toxic fumes, heat and evacuation problems. In case of impact, you should leave the plane within ninety seconds - book your seat by the aisle, not by the window, and as close as possible to an exit (within five rows distance) so that you can move quickly to the exit.

Always seat your family together, in order to save time when looking for them after a crash. When flying, it is essential to listen to the safety briefing and carefully read the safety briefing cards; practice the release of your seat belt and learn where the exits are in your plane; learn and practice the brace position as it protects your body.

Frequent fliers could also consider carrying a mini-respirator to provide a few valuable minutes of safe breathing in the unlikely event of an accident.

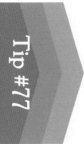

Tip #77

▶ Select seats near the emergency exits
▶ Be alert during take-off and landing
▶ Keep your seat belt fastened at all times

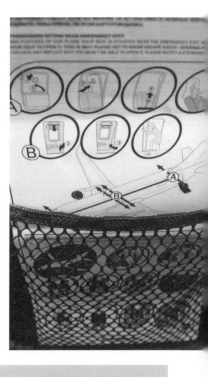

Information

Deadly Stupidity: What NOT To Do in an Emergency
Ask the Pilot - https://go22.uk/askthepilot

Bureau of Aircraft Accidents Archives (B3A) -
https://go22.uk/b3a
Includes death rates per year and per operator

Will wearing a seatbelt on a plane save your life?
The Telegraph - https://go22.uk/seatbelt

Products

MSA miniSCAPE Escape respirator - £37 (~US$48)
Frontline Safety - https://go22.uk/miniscape

Global Fatal Accident Review 2002-2011
Civil Aviation Authority - https://go22.uk/rp0871
Approach, landing and go-around phases accounted for 47% of all fatal accidents

An analysis of exit availability, exit usage and passenger exit selection behaviour exhibited during actual aviation accidents
The Aeronautical Journal - https://go22.uk/rp0872

COST: ●● ○ ○ ○   EASE: ●●●● ○   IMPACT: ●● ○ ○ ○

Cars - autonomous emergency braking

Autonomous Emergency Braking (AEB) is a safety technology aimed at reducing the risk of car crashes by maximising the braking capacity of the vehicle. Compared to normal emergency braking, AEB has the ability to start braking the vehicle sooner than a driver could possibly do, and optimising the brake pressure. Thus, AEB reduces the reaction period in a potential crash. A study, that used police-reported crashes, between 2010 and 2014, in Sweden, statistically demonstrated that the use of AEB systems resulted in a 35-41% reduction in rear-end crashes.

A recent study calculated the potential of Autonomous Emergency Braking (AEB) in reducing fatal and injury crashes by simulating real crash data from South Australia. Through computational programs and analysis, AEB systems were estimated to reduce fatal crashes by 20-27% and injury crashes by 27-37%.

There are three categories of AEB, the low speed system, which is designed to detect vehicles in front of a car to prevent non-life-threatening crashes; the higher speed system, which has a long-range radar that scans up to 200 m at higher speeds; and the pedestrian system, which detects the presence of pedestrian movement to minimize the risk of collision.

Car manufacturers have different names for their AEB systems. For instance, Mercedes-Benz calls it the PRE-SAFE Brake, Audi calls it the Pre Sense Plus, Ford has the Active City Stop, and Honda has the Collision Mitigation Braking System.

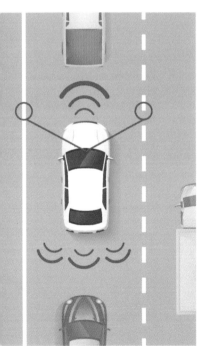

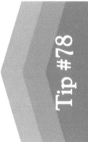

▷ Choose a car with an AEB system
▷ Look for other features such as lane-departure and blind-spot warnings
▷ Retrofit the latest technology to your existing car

Tip #78

Information
Cars With Advanced Safety Systems
Consumer Reports - https://go22.uk/carsafety

Use the latest technology to update your old car
RAC - https://go22.uk/cartech

Products
Mio Mivue 792 WIFI Pro - £159 (~US$205)
Dash cam with lane departure & collision warning systems, plus a driver fatigue alert - https://go22.uk/miomivue

Potential Benefits of AEB Based on In-Depth Crash Reconstruction and Simulation
International Technical Conference on the Enhanced Safety of Vehicles - https://go22.uk/rp0661
AEB systems can potentially reduce fatal crashes by up to 20-27%

The Injury Crash Reduction of Low-speed Autonomous Emergency Braking on Passenger Cars
International Research Council on the Biomechanics of Injury - https://go22.uk/rp0662
The use of AEB systems resulted to 35-41% reduction in rear-end crashes

COST: ● ● ● ● ●   EASE: ● ● ● ● ●   IMPACT: ● ● ● ● ●

Car safety ratings

It is easy to feel safe when cocooned in the metal cage of a car, however, in the US alone the equivalent of two 747 airplanes full of passengers die on the roads every week. This is only overlooked by the media, because the deaths happen a few at a time.

Other tips in this book suggest ways of avoiding accidents with technology and staying alert, but what if the worst case happens and you are involved in an accident? What is the best way of improving your chance of surviving? This is where car safety ratings are crucial. The advice is to buy a car with the highest safety rating that you can afford.

The Euro NCAP is a measure of crashworthiness used for cars in Europe using a five-star safety rating system. The safety rating is calculated by testing vehicles in multiple real-life accident scenarios to determine the likelihood of death or injury to the car occupants and other road users.

Studies that correlate actual police reports to NCAP ratings have shown that compared to 2-star cars, 3- and 4-star cars have a 30% lower risk of a fatality in a crash, and that jumps to a 68% reduction in 5-star cars.

In the US, the National Highway Traffic Safety Administration (NHTSA) assesses vehicles using a 5-Star Safety Ratings system and uniquely includes a rollover resistance test.

▷ Choose the highest safety-rated car that
you can afford

Tip #79

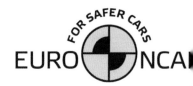

★★★★★

★★★★☆

★★★☆☆

★★☆☆☆

★☆☆☆☆

Organisations
Euro NCAP - https://go22.uk/euroncap
European car safety performance assessment programme

NHTSA - https://go22.uk/nhtsa
Responsible for keeping people safe on America's roadways

Information
The cheapest new cars with 5 stars for safety
Motoring Research - https://go22.uk/cheap5stars

Comparison Between Euro NCAP Test Results and Real-World Crash Data
Traffic Injury Prevention - https://go22.uk/rp0351
Five-star cars have a 68% lower risk of fatal injuries during collisions

How Do Euro NCAP Results Correlate with Real-Life Injury Risks?
Traffic Injury Prevention - https://go22.uk/rp0352
Three or four-star cars are approximately 30% safer than 2-star cars

COST: ●●●●○   EASE: ●●●●●   IMPACT: ●●●○○

Cycling safety

Whereas cycling has been shown to increase longevity through an increase in cardiovascular fitness, it is also an activity that represents a risk of an accident, including potentially severe injury to the head, brain, and face. Injuries sustained from biking can be fatal, with 102 reported cyclist deaths in the UK in 2016.

One of the most simple and effective means to minimise the risk of serious head injury while cycling is by wearing a helmet. Cyclists who end up in the emergency room for accidental injury are almost overwhelmingly people who were not wearing a helmet. Helmets lead to dramatic reductions in the risk of injury to the head, face and brain, and significantly reduce the risk of fatal injury, with some studies showing a reduction of almost a third.

There is some evidence that the statistics are more complicated. Although wearing a helmet reduces the chance of injury in an accident, the chance of having an accident actually increases when wearing a helmet. This is because both the cyclist and other road users take fewer precautions. However, for now, the general advice seems to be that it is safer to wear a properly-fitted helmet.

When buying a helmet, make sure it is safety certified. For example, EN1078 helmets are designed to withstand a head impact on a kerb when falling from one metre at 12mph.

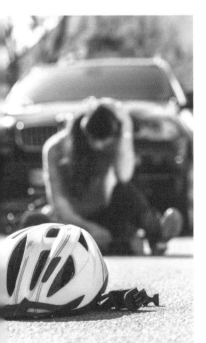

▷ Wear a safety-standard marked helmet whenever you ride your bike
▷ Be careful when passing vehicles on the inside of the road
▷ Look properly when entering and crossing main roads

Tip #80

Information

Cycle Helmet Safety Standards Explained
Global Cycling Network (YouTube) -
https://go22.uk/cyclehelmets

University ranks helmets for safety
Bike Radar - https://go22.uk/helmetsafety
In Virginia Tech's testing, cost did not predict performance. Awards star ratings to 30 popular helmets.

Bicycle Helmet Efficacy: a Meta-analysis
Accident Analysis & Prevention - https://go22.uk/rp0781
Wearing a helmet significantly reduces risk of head and brain injuries, as well as the risk of death

Cycling Accidents - Road Safety Factsheet
Royal Society for the Prevention of Accidents - https://go22.uk/rp0782

COST: ● ● ● ● ●   EASE: ● ● ● ● ●   IMPACT: ● ● ● ○ ○

Driving while alert

The Department for Transport reported that 65% of the car accidents, recorded in 2016, in the UK, were caused by driver or rider error or poor reaction. This includes failing to look properly, judging another driver's speed incorrectly, or poor turns and manoeuvres. It makes sense, then, that the best way to keep safe while driving is to minimise one's risk of driving errors.

It has been clearly demonstrated that driving while drowsy diminishes human judgment and reaction times. When compared with drowsy drivers, drivers who are alert or relaxed and well-rested have a 19% reduced risk of a car crash resulting in death or injury.

Beyond the obvious things such as keeping a well-maintained vehicle and wearing a seatbelt, maintaining alertness while driving is perhaps the single most effective way to drive safely. Drinking tea or coffee, listening to the radio, and taking frequent breaks while driving long distances will all help you keep yourself safe on the road. Of course, the most important thing, though, is to only drive when you are alert and have had adequate sleep.

Tip #81

▶ Drive only when alert and well-rested
▶ Take a break when driving for extended periods
▶ Undertake advanced driver training to improve your skills and awareness

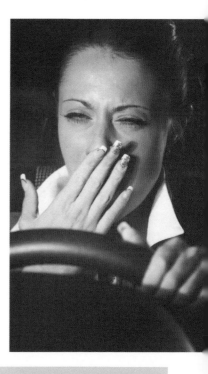

Organisations
IAM RoadSmart (formerly Institute of Advanced Motorists) - https://go22.uk/roadsmart
Provides advanced driver training courses that can lead to cheaper insurance

Products
StopSleep - £179 (~US$230) - https://go22.uk/stopsleep
Analyses the skin's electrodermal activity and sounds an alarm when cerebral activity drops

Samsung Copilot - free - https://go22.uk/copilot
Smartwatch app measures your state of alertness

Road accidents and safety statistics
UK Department for Transport - https://go22.uk/rp0851

Drowsiness, counter-measures to drowsiness, and the risk of a motor vehicle crash
Injury Prevention - https://go22.uk/rp0852
This study shows the reduction of crash risk associated with a variety of interventions to increase general alertness

COST: ● ● ● ● ●   EASE: ● ● ● ● ○   IMPACT: ● ● ○ ○ ○

Holiday deaths

Travelling abroad is a rewarding experience; immersing oneself into a new culture and having adventures, as well as relaxing. But it is important not to forget about staying safe. In 2014, 3,670 British nationals died while abroad, which means one in every sixteen thousand trips overseas resulted in a death – making a foreign trip six times more dangerous than a single parachute jump!

The countries with the highest rate of British national deaths are Thailand, the Philippines, Cyprus and Switzerland, although the highest number of tourist murders are in Pakistan, Jamaica and America.

All of these death rates are low and can be further minimised by taking a few precautions to prevent deaths related to theft and assault. Choose a hotel in a good neighbourhood and reserve an upper level room. Take a small doorstop in case the lock doesn't work and buy a self-defence spray (where legal) as a backup. Always lock your hotel room and close the window.

Don't flaunt possessions and large amounts of money - use the hotel safe. Avoid walking alone at night, and only use licensed taxis, preferably arranged for via hotels and restaurants. Holiday means having fun, but moderate your drinking - alcohol slows down reactions and affects judgement. Don't leave food and drinks unattended in public places, to prevent anyone slipping drugs into them.

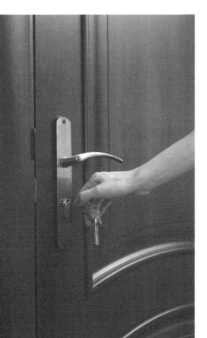

▷ Check the FCO website before you go – do not travel if advised against

▷ Take extra precautions in high risk destinations

▷ Always pay attention to personal safety and room security

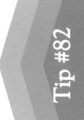

Tip #82

Information
Foreign and Commonwealth Office travel advice - https://go22.uk/fcotravel
Detailed information and up-to-date assessment of security and risks by country

5 Easy Ways to Secure Your Hotel Room
Trip Savvy - https://go22.uk/securehotel
Cheap, Portable Safety When You Travel

Products
Travel Safety Gadgets – from £2 (~US$2)
Gap Year Travel Store - https://go22.uk/gapyear
Door locks, bag protectors, and safety alarms

Helping British Nationals Abroad 2014/15
reign and Commonwealth Office - https://go22.uk/rp0861
Official statistics registered 3,670 deaths of British nationals abroad in 2014/2015 and 4,110 cases in 2013/2014

COST: ● ● ● ● ●   EASE: ● ● ● ● ○   IMPACT: ● ● ○ ○ ○

Motorbikes

Motorcyclists travel 2.8 billion miles annually in UK. The number is impressive, but unfortunately so are the statistics of casualties. In 2016, 319 motorcyclists were killed on the roads, and 5,553 were seriously injured, according to the Department For Transport.

Motorcycle riders are over sixty times more likely to be killed in traffic accidents than car occupants. Most accidents occur at junctions and in rural areas. The Road Safety Observatory states that half of deaths and serious injuries to motorcyclists occurred at a junction where another vehicle pulled out in front of the motorcyclist. However, one in four did not involve another vehicle and were often caused by the rider misjudging a bend.

Although younger riders have more accidents, they tend to be less serious because they are on motorbikes with smaller engines. There is a higher risk of death in the over thirties where the engine size is over 500 cc.

Stay safe by following some basic rules: ride a motorcycle within your ability, wear the right gear, including high visibility elements. And of course, always wear a helmet – they reduce the risk of death by 42%.

Tip #83

▶ Don't ride a motorbike
▶ If you must, always wear a helmet
▶ Ride within your ability and keep some safety contingency going into bends

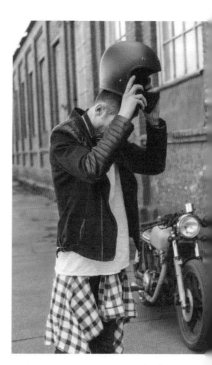

Information
Motorcycle safety advice
British Motorcyclists Federation -
https://go22.uk/bmfsafety
Including how to avoid the 5 most common motorcycle accidents

Motorcycle Helmet Standards Explained
Ultimate Motorcycling -
https://go22.uk/motohelmets
Detailed explanation of DOT, ECE 22.05 & Snell

The five key skills that new riders need to master
Motor Cycle News - https://go22.uk/mcnskills

Riders - Motorcyclists - Detailed Review
Road Safety Observatory - https://go22.uk/rp0881
This synthesis was compiled during July 2011, and updated in January 2017

Helmets for preventing injury in motorcycle riders
Cochrane Systematic Review - https://go22.uk/rp0882
Motorcycle helmets reduced the risk of death by 42%

COST: ● ● ● ● ●　　　EASE: ● ● ● ● ○　　　IMPACT: ● ● ● ○ ○

Blood donation

As well as the amazing feeling of being able to save someone's life, blood donation also has physical benefits for the donor. Most of the benefits are related to iron which is an essential element in the human body, involved in a wide variety of metabolic processes, including oxygen transport and DNA synthesis.

While iron is a vital to health, too much iron can lead to higher risk of cardiovascular ailments, liver disease, diabetes, and cancer. High iron levels constrict blood vessels, reduce blood flow, and oxidize cholesterol which in turn harden arteries and increase the risk of atherosclerosis and heart attacks.

By donating blood, not only do iron levels decrease, but blood viscosity is also reduced which improves the circulatory system. In addition, excess iron can reduce insulin sensitivity, so blood donations may lower the risk of diabetes. What's more, many infectious agents require iron to survive and grow, so donating may reduce the occurrence of general illnesses.

Most people who are generally fit and well are able to donate blood, though there are some exclusions, such as those who have had a recent operation or are on certain medications, so always check before donating.

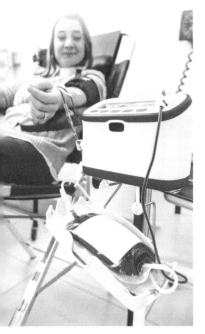

▷ Donate blood at least once a year

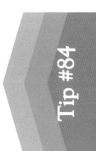

Tip #84

Information
Frequently Asked Questions on Blood Donation
World Health Organization –
https://go22.uk/bloodfaq

Organisations
Blood donation centres:
England - https://go22.uk/bloodeng
Scotland - https://go22.uk/bloodsco
Wales - https://go22.uk/bloodwal
Northern Ireland - https://go22.uk/bloodnir
United States - https://go22.uk/bloodusa
Canada - https://go22.uk/bloodcan

Blood donation and blood donor mortality after adjustment for a healthy donor effect
Transfusion - https://go22.uk/rp0991
High frequency of blood donation is associated with a lower risk of mortality rate

Improving health profile of blood donors as a consequence of transfusion safety efforts
Transfusion - https://go22.uk/rp0992
Blood donors enjoy better than average health, with reduced risk of mortality & cancer incidence

COST: ● ● ● ○ ○   EASE: ● ● ● ○ ○   IMPACT: ● ● ○ ○ ○

Cryotherapy

Cryotherapy is a treatment for inflammatory conditions such as stiffness and swelling. As chronic inflammation is a biomarker of ageing, anything that reduces it will have a beneficial effect on ageing.

Whole-body cryotherapy (WBC) is the exposure of the entire body to very low temperatures, typically between -80 °C and -160 °C (-110 to – 260 °F) in order to initiate a physiological response. The therapy usually involves walking into a fridge-like cryochamber wearing little more than your underwear and a headband to prevent frostbite. Cryotherapy is popular amongst elite athletes and the use of cryochambers is considered safe when done correctly. Extreme temperatures are involved so it should never be undertaken unaccompanied.

Its main effects are on the motor system and it is used to cure inflammatory musculoskeletal diseases, such as rheumatoid arthritis, osteoarthritis, and chronic inflammation of the cervical spine. Cryotherapy has been shown to increase active muscle power and reduce oedema which results in a wider range of motion in the inflamed joints. It is also used for treating depression disorders because it induces the production of endorphins which relieve stress.

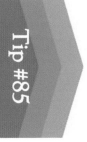

Tip #85

▷ Have an occasional cryotherapy session
▷ NOTE: cryotherapy should be avoided by people who have a heart condition or issues with blood pressure

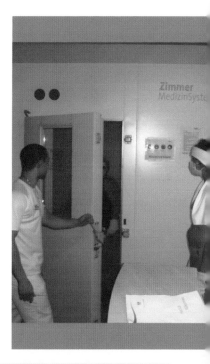

Information
17 Proven Benefits of Whole Body Cryotherapy + Side Effects
Self Hacked - https://go22.uk/cryo17

Products
BMI Hendon Hospital - https://go22.uk/bmicryo
£50 for a whole-body cryotherapy session

Chris Moody Sports Therapy and Injury Rehabilitation Centre - https://go22.uk/chrismoody
Dual chamber fits 2 people for £53 for 3 minutes

Do sessions of cryostimulation have influence on white blood cell count ... in healthy men?
European Journal of Applied Physiology - https://go22.uk/rp0831
Extremely low temperatures used have mobilization effect on immunological system

Whole-Body Cryostimulation as Effective Method of Reducing Oxidative Stress in Healthy Men
Advances in Clinical and Experimental Medicine - https://go22.uk/rp0832
Statistically significant decrease in concentrations of most of the parameters of oxidative stress

COST: ● ● ● ● ○   EASE: ● ● ● ● ○   IMPACT: ● ● ● ○ ○

Flu vaccination

Many people think of the flu as just a bad cold. But seasonal influenza can be very serious with severe symptoms including fever, muscle and joint pain, and headache. Although most people recover, without treatment, in three to seven days, an estimated 14,000 people die from flu each year in the US, and a similar number in Europe.

The best way to prevent avoid the flu is with an annual vaccination. The influenza virus is constantly changing which means that resistance to the previous flu season may not have any impact on the following year. It also means that the particular structure of the virus is hard to predict, hence the vaccine's effectiveness varies between about 20-60% each year. However, as well as reducing the chances of catching the flu, a vaccination also reduces the symptoms in the people who do catch it. Once caught, adults are up to five times more likely to die of influenza if they're unvaccinated.

In industrialised countries the highest risk of deaths associated with influenza is among people age 65 or older, nevertheless, all ages are vulnerable so it is recommended that everyone gets a jab. Also, a recent study found that vaccine effectiveness falls steadily over time so it's better not to get a flu shot too early in the season, but still generally before the end of October.

Some people report mild side-effects from the vaccine injection, though some of these experiences will be because the injection coincided with a naturally occurring infection. It is not possible to get the flu from a flu vaccination.

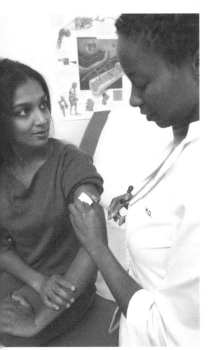

▷ Get a flu jab every year – whatever age you are

▷ See a doctor if flu symptoms don't improve after seven days

Tip #86

Information

Influenza - What you need to know
BMJ - https://go22.uk/flu2know

Dispelling deadly myths about the flu vaccine
Washington Post - https://go22.uk/flumyths

Products

Boots Winter Flu Jab Service - £12.99, or free on NHS if eligible - https://go22.uk/bootsflujab

Where to Get Cheap or Free Flu Shots (USA)
20 Something Finance - https://go22.uk/cheapflu
He's got on the phone and done the research!

End-of-season influenza vaccine effectiveness in adults and children, United Kingdom, 2016/17
Eurosurveillance - https://go22.uk/rp1311
Across all age groups including children, the flu vaccine prevented 39.8% of flu cases

Intraseason waning of influenza vaccine protection: Evidence from 2011-12 through 2014-15
Clinical Infectious Diseases - https://go22.uk/rp1312
Maximum vaccine effectiveness was observed shortly after vaccination

COST: ● ● ● ● ● EASE: ● ● ● ● ● IMPACT: ● ● ● ● ● ●

Hyperbaric oxygen therapy

Hyperbaric Oxygen Therapy (HBOT) aims to make more oxygen available to the body's tissues. This is done by breathing pure oxygen in a high-pressure environment. HBOT typically involves breathing oxygen at twice atmospheric pressure (in a special pressure vessel) for one to two hours. Painless and efficient, HBOT is approved for the treatment of many different diseases, such as non-healing wounds, brain injuries, stroke, burns, and carbon monoxide poisoning.

The mechanism behind its healing power is that HBOT helps to widen the body's blood vessels, improving circulation and stimulating the formation of new blood capillaries to oxygen-starved areas. Like a domino effect, increased oxygen supply reduces pain and turns off inflammation and cell death, which in turn prevents infections and triggers the body's natural healing process.

Furthermore, HBOT could be used to prevent many degenerative diseases, as it increases the production of stem cells and promotes the natural defence activity of white blood cells.

NOTE: this is not to be confused with oxygen bars which involves breathing extra oxygen at normal atmospheric pressure. There is no evidence that this has any long-term beneficial effects. Red blood cells leaving the lungs are already almost 100% saturated with oxygen. In contrast, at the higher pressures involved in HBOT, the blood plasma is used to transport additional oxygen to the cells.

Tip #87

▷ Undertake a series of hyperbaric oxygen therapy

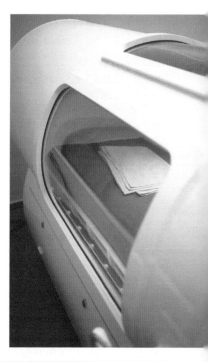

Information
What is hyperbaric oxygen therapy good for?
Medical News Today - https://go22.uk/hbotgood

Products
Find a chamber
Hyperbaric Oxygen Treatment Trust -
https://go22.uk/hbotfind

Hyperbaric Oxygen Therapy Centre -
https://go22.uk/hbotcentre
5 x 1 hour sessions = £750 (US$980)

HBOT increases insulin sensitivity in overweight men with and without type 2 diabetes
Diving and Hyperbaric Medicine - https://go22.uk/rp0791
HBOT increased peripheral insulin sensitivity increase was associated with reduction in TNF

Adaptive protection against the induction of oxidative DNA damage after HBOT
Carcinogenesis - https://go22.uk/rp0792
HBO treatment is well protected against the in vitro induction of DNA damage by H2O2

COST: ● ● ○ ○ ○   EASE: ● ● ● ● ○   IMPACT: ● ● ○ ○ ○

Massage

Massage therapy is one of the oldest forms of health treatment, dating back 3,000 years, according to Chinese records.

Massage improves overall health. Its wide-ranging effects include lowering blood pressure, reducing pain and swelling, increased alertness, and also enhancing the body's immune function. As well as its physical benefits, massage reduces stress, reduce depression and has been found to alleviate migraine headaches.

There are many types of massage, with Swedish or therapeutic massage being the most widely available. A typical session lasts thirty to sixty minutes. Variations of these basic styles include the use of hot stones to relieve more muscle tension by adding extra heat to the body, and also aromatherapy which uses essential oils (plant extracts such as lavender and sandalwood) to add an emotional healing component to the massage.

There are no formal qualifications required to be a massage therapist, so it is a good idea to check for professional memberships, qualifications, and ongoing training commitments when looking for a masseur.

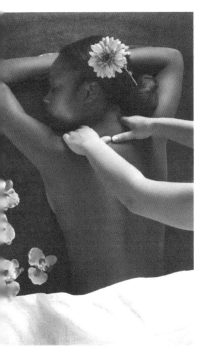

▷ Have a massage once a month

Tip #88

Information
Massage Therapy Styles and Health Benefits
WebMD - https://go22.uk/massageben

How to Find a Good Massage Therapist
PainScience.com - https://go22.uk/findmassage

Products
The Complete Body Massage Course (book)
Nicola Stewart - https://go22.uk/bodymassage

Swedish Massage: A Systematic Review of its Physical and Psychological Benefits
Advances In Mind-body Medicine - https://go22.uk/rp0581
Shown beneficial effects in multiple populations, use in disease prevention highly recommended

Effects of Swedish massage on blood pressure
Complementary Therapies in Clinical Practice - https://go22.uk/rp0582
Back, neck and chest massage decreases systolic as well as diastolic blood pressure

COST: ● ● ● ○ ○   EASE: ● ● ● ○ ○   IMPACT: ● ● ● ● ○

Metformin

Metformin is an excellent treatment against diabetes - it inhibits glucose production and increases glucose uptake. It is safe, with very well-known activity and low toxicity.

Interestingly, there is now significant evidence to indicate that metformin can increase life expectancy and reduce the risk of cancer and cardiovascular disease in mice and, to a certain extent, in humans.

Although used as a diabetes drug for over 60 years, metformin was labelled as the new anti-ageing drug by the world's press when, in 2017, it became the subject of a human clinical trial to investigate its effects on the biology of ageing. The study is examining whether metformin affects the cellular processes associated with age-related conditions, such as inflammation, oxidative damage, diminished autophagy, and cell senescence. In particular, it will look into whether it restores the gene expression profile of older adults with impaired glucose tolerance to that of young healthy subjects. Another aim of the trial is to persuade the FDA to classify ageing as an "indication" for which treatments can be approved.

Metformin is now out of patent and hence available (via prescription) cheaply as a generic drug, as well as under common brand names (e.g. Fortamet, Glucophage, Glumetza, Riomet). One biological mechanism through which metformin works is by activating an enzyme, called AMPK, that boosts cellular energy. Therefore, while waiting for metformin approval, taking an AMPK activator may have similar results.

Tip #89

▶ Ask your doctor whether you are a candidate for metformin

▶ Alternatively, include an AMPK activator in your daily supplement regime

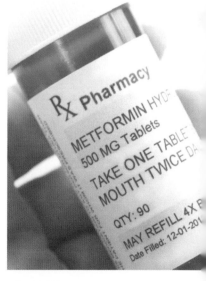

Information
Drugs.com - https://go22.uk/drugsmetf

Metformin in Longevity Study (MILES)
Clinical trial details - https://go22.uk/metfmiles

Products
AMPK Metabolic Activator
Life Extension - https://go22.uk/ampkle

Can people with type 2 diabetes live longer than those without?
Diabetes, Obesity and Metabolism - https://go22.uk/rp0101
Metformin monotherapy patients had longer survival than matched, non-diabetic controls

Association of metformin use with cancer incidence and mortality: A meta-analysis
Cancer Epidemiology - https://go22.uk/rp0102
Metformin reduces the incidence of overall cancer by 27%

COST: ●●● ○ ○   EASE: ●● ○ ○ ○   IMPACT: ●● ○ ○ ○

Radiation hormesis

High levels of radiation are most definitely dangerous, resulting in cancer and even death within weeks at extremely high doses. However, low level background radiation occurs naturally (e.g. from rocks, soil and cosmic rays) and the body has evolved repair mechanisms to compensate for this.

Hormesis is when an organism's response to a small exposure to a stressor (e.g. cold temperatures, toxins) overcompensates for the damage caused, and therefore has an overall positive effect. These hormetic effects have been observed in response to physical stressors in plants and simple animals as well as in humans.

Radiation hormesis was overlooked for decades because of the acceptance of the linear no-threshold model. This model extrapolates the proven harm from high levels of radiation back down to very low levels, even though limited research has been done below levels of 100 millisievert (mSv) per year. In fact, studies on some populations that have been exposed to low levels of radiation have suggested the opposite. For example, in the 1980s recycled nuclear reactor steel was accidentally used in the construction of 2,000 apartments in Taiwan, resulting in long-term exposure to 10,000 people. Surprisingly, the cancer rates in these people was significantly below average.

Radiation hormesis is available as a health treatment at several spas, which are built underground in high radon areas. Typically, a course of ten sessions will result in an exposure of 2 mSv. For comparison, a full-body CT scan administers 10 mSv, and the annual exposure for a long-haul airline crew is 9 mSv.

▷ **Make an occasional visit to a radon therapy spa**

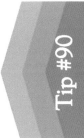

Tip #90

Information
Could Small Amounts of Radiation Be Good For You? It's Complicated
Discover magazine - https://go22.uk/smallrad

Products
Free Enterprise Radon Mine - https://go22.uk/ferhm
Montana, USA - US$8.00 per hour

Gastein Healing Gallery - https://go22.uk/gastein
Austria – 68 Euros (US$75) per session

ACURADON - https://go22.uk/acuradon
Germany - 29 Euros (US$32) per session

Nuclear shipyard worker study: a large cohort exposed to low-dose-rate gamma radiation
International Journal of Low Radiation - https://go22.uk/rp0071
Long term exposure to gamma radiation significantly decrease Standardized mortality

Potential Solutions in Radiation Hormesis
Journal of Cancer Research Updates - https://go22.uk/rp0072
Low dose radiation elevates immune response, may reduce rather than increase risk of cancer

COST: ● ● ● ○ ○   EASE: ● ● ○ ○ ○   IMPACT: ● ● ○ ○ ○

Rapamycin

Rapamycin (also known as sirolimus) is produced by bacteria native to the soil of Easter Island in the Pacific Ocean. Initially used as an antifungal agent, researchers have discovered other interesting properties of rapamycin such as its being an immunosuppressant. It is now regularly used in tissue transplant procedures, particularly because of its low kidney toxicity.

Rapamycin has also been shown to act as an inhibitor of cell senescence and to increase lifespan in animal studies. In a recent study, an improvement in the cardiac function of dogs was observed after just ten weeks of rapamycin treatment. Excitingly, it appears to have a significant effect on lifespan (10% longer in mice) even when taken at a late age.

It is likely that some form of rapamycin (known as rapalogs, e.g. everolimus) will eventually become available to the general public with recommended dosages guided by further human trials. However, although it is rumoured that some doctors and scientists are already self-prescribing rapamycin, it should only be taken under proper medical supervision.

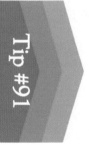

Tip #91

▶ Consult a doctor about being prescribed rapamycin

Information

Rapamycin – the Easter Island drug that extends lifespan of old mice
Discover magazine - https://go22.uk/rapamice

U.S. Doc Prescribing Anti-Aging Cocktail To Seniors
Longevity Facts - https://go22.uk/aacocktail

New tricks from old dogs join the fight against ageing
Nature - https://go22.uk/rapatrick

Rapamycin may slow aging
The Aesthetic Channel - https://go22.uk/rapaslow

rapamycin

TORC1 inhibition enhances immune function and reduces infections in the elderly
Science Translational Medicine - https://go22.uk/rp0801
Low-dose TORC1 inhibitor therapy in elderly humans decreased the incidence of all infections

mTOR inhibition improves immune function in the elderly
Science Translational Medicine - https://go22.uk/rp0802
mTOR inhibition may have beneficial effects on immunosenescence in the elderly

COST: ● ○ ○ ○ ○   EASE: ● ○ ○ ○ ○   IMPACT: ● ● ● ● ●

Senescent cells

Cells that have lost their ability to function and divide usually commit cellular suicide (apoptosis), in order to be recycled and to make room for new cells. This mechanism plays an important role in preventing malfunctioning cells from becoming cancerous. However, sometimes these cells don't die, instead becoming senescent. They remain in place reducing the performance of the tissue and also secreting inflammatory proteins (SASP) that impair the function of surrounding cells.

Senescent cells accumulate over time, and by middle-age they start to make an increasing contribution to many age-related diseases, including type 2 diabetes and atherosclerosis. One approach to reversing this damage is to use senolytics – drugs that either induce senescent cells to complete apoptosis or encourage the immune system to kill them. There has been some particularly interesting research, recently, on the use of senolytics in mice. In a 2016 study, treatment with a senolytic resulted in an average 25% life extension even though it was not applied to the mice until the equivalent of 58 human-years old.

Several companies have raised investment to develop senolytics. Although not yet available for prescription, several drug candidates are entering human clinical trials for which some people may be eligible.

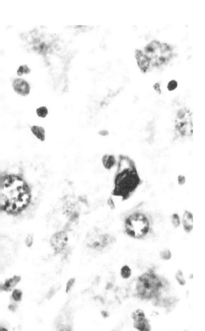

▷ If possible, sign up to human clinical trial for senolytics
▷ Monitor senolytic developers for news and product releases

Tip #92

Information
To stay young, kill zombie cells
Nature - https://go22.uk/zombiecells

Race to develop senescent cell clearance therapies
Signals - https://go22.uk/race2sen

Products
The following companies are developing senolytics:
ANTOXERENE - https://go22.uk/antoxerene
Cleara - https://go22.uk/cleara
Oisin Biotechnologies - https://go22.uk/oisinbio
UNITY Biotechnology* - https://go22.uk/unitybio
*currently recruiting for human clinical trial

Cellular Senescence: The Sought or the Unwanted?
Trends in Molecular Medicine - https://go22.uk/rp0251
Senolytics are effective in extending healthspan, reducing frailty, improving stem cell function

Naturally occurring p16Ink4a-positive cells shorten healthy lifespan
Nature - https://go22.uk/rp0252
Therapeutic removal of senescent cells may be an attractive approach to extend healthy lifespan

COST: ● ● ● ● ○   EASE: ● ● ● ○ ○   IMPACT: ● ● ● ○ ○

Statins

Statins are a group of medicines that can fight cardiovascular diseases (CVD) – the world's leading cause of death. They can even prevent the first heart attack or stroke in normally healthy people and prevent about 80,000 heart attacks more generally in the UK every year.

Statins reduce the level of LDL (bad cholesterol) by blocking an enzyme crucial to the body's manufacture of cholesterol. This, in turn, helps prevent the build-up of fatty plaques in blood vessels, preventing further blockage in blood vessels and reducing the risk of heart attacks.

Besides being effective in lowering cholesterol, statins also have potent anti-inflammatory and antioxidant properties. Moreover, statin use has been found to have a beneficial effect in treating and preventing many infections.

UK guidelines were updated in 2014, to recommend that anyone with a higher than 10% risk of developing CVD over ten years should be offered atorvastatin (a specific statin) as a preventative treatment. However, as with all drugs, statins may have side effects so always be aware of these.

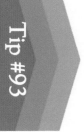

Tip #93

▸ Talk to your doctor about a statin prescription even if you only have a low risk of cardiovascular disease
▸ Statins are not recommended for pregnant women or those with liver disease

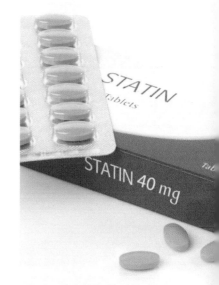

Information

NICE recommends wider use of statins for prevention of CVD
National Institute for Health and Care Excellence - https://go22.uk/nicestatins

Statin side effects: Weigh the benefits and risks
Mayo Clinic - https://go22.uk/statinside

Generic vs. brand-name statins
Harvard Health Letter - https://go22.uk/genstatins

Lowering LDL cholesterol with statin therapy in people at low risk of vascular disease
Lancet - https://go22.uk/rp1041
Statins reduce LDL cholesterol and prevent vascular events

Statins for the primary prevention of cardiovascular disease
Cochrane Database of Systematic Reviews - https://go22.uk/rp1042
Reduction in all-cause mortality found with no excess of adverse events in non-CVD people

COST: ● ● ○ ○ ○   EASE: ● ● ○ ○ ○   IMPACT: ● ● ● ● ●

Stem Cells

Stem cells are those that are able to divide to create copies of themselves, and uniquely, to develop into specific types of cells (e.g. heart, skin, blood). They are the body's building and repair machinery. Most adult stem cells are only able to create a few types of tissues, however embryonic stem cells (ESCs), which are found in early-stage embryos, are pluripotent and able to differentiate into any of 200 cell types. Significant effort has gone into creating induced pluripotent stem cells (iPSCs), which are normal cells that have been genetically reprogrammed to behave more like ESCs.

Treatments using stem cells have already been established for arthritis and some blood cancers. One clinical trial is using patients' own stem cells to improve their chances of recovery after a heart attack. More potential treatments are in early research, such as using stem cells to grow new bladder muscle and retina cells.

Unfortunately, stem cells also age and decrease in number over time. It is possible to bank some of them now, so that they are available (and in a more youthful state) should you need them for treatment in the future. As well as being used for a growing list of conditions, it is likely that in the future stem cells could be used to enhance the immune system and turn back the ageing clock.

Although most stem cell banks specialise in storing ESCs from cord blood, or youthful stem cells from children's milk teeth, some offer a service of extracting adult stem cells from a small fat sample. By the time they are needed, further medical advances should make it possible to revert them to iPSCs suitable for a myriad of treatments.

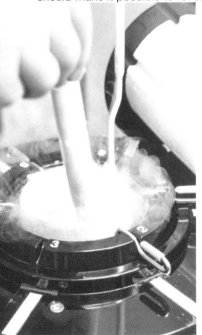

▷ Bank some of your stem cells for future treatments

▷ If you have an existing condition, check if a stem cell therapy clinical trial is available

Tip #94

Information
Stem cells: What they are and what they do
Mayo Clinic - https://go22.uk/whatarestemcells

Search for a stem cell clinical trial for your disease
Knoepfler Lab - https://go22.uk/search4stem

Products
Smart Cells - https://go22.uk/smartcells
Adult stem cell storage - £1,995 + £95/year
Celltex - https://go22.uk/celltex
Adult stem cell storage - US$6,350 + $150/year
Spire Healthcare - https://go22.uk/spirestem
Treatment for arthritis and cartilage regeneration

Stem cell therapy for chronic ischaemic heart disease and congestive heart failure
Cochrane Database of Systematic Reviews - https://go22.uk/rp0261
Treatment with adult stem cells reduces mortality, improves left ventricular ejection fraction

Clinical Outcomes of Transplanted Modified Marrow-Derived Mesenchymal Stem Cells in Stroke
Stroke - https://go22.uk/rp0262
Intracerebral stem cell transplant of SB623 cells is safe and associated with improvement

COST: ● ○ ○ ○ ○   EASE: ● ○ ○ ○ ○   IMPACT: ● ● ● ● ●

Young blood

As well as red blood cells (that carry oxygen) and white blood cells (the immune system), blood is also composed of plasma which contains, among other substances, proteins, glucose, clotting factors and hormones. One function of this mixture is to regulate the metabolism. As the balance of proteins in blood plasma changes over time, so does the functioning of the body.

Parabiosis experiments (where the circulatory systems are artificially joined together) in mice have demonstrated rejuvenation of older mice when connected to younger mice. Further research is being undertaken to determine whether the effect is because of positive factors in the young blood, or the dilution of negative factors in the old blood, or perhaps a combination of both.

A human clinical trial of youthful blood plasma injections has been undertaken by a US company called Ambrosia. Although they have not published results yet, they claim the treatment has led to improvements in the biomarkers related to cancer, Alzheimer's disease and heart disease. No prices have been announced yet, though participation in the clinical trial cost $8,000 so it is likely to be in that ball park.

Meanwhile, Dr.s Irina and Michael Conboy at University of California, Berkeley, are researching ways to filter out negative factors from old blood to make it young again. Their targets are the inhibitory proteins (such as TGF-B1) that impair tissue repair. They are developing a blood filtering device (called NextGen apheresis) for people to use at a clinic once every few months.

Tip #95

▶ Join Ambrosia's waiting list for young plasma treatments

▶ If you have Alzheimer's disease, consider joining a clinical trial being run by Alkahest

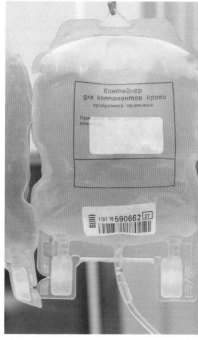

Information

Rejuvenating Old Brains with Young Blood
YouTube - https://go22.uk/youngmice
Watch old mice perform as if young in maze tests

Can young blood really rejuvenate the old?
The Economist - https://go22.uk/youngeco

Products

Ambrosia - https://go22.uk/ambrosia
Will provide blood plasma treatments in New York

Alkahest - https://go22.uk/alkahest
Currently running human clinical trials

Rejuvenation of aged progenitor cells by exposure to a young systemic environment
Nature - https://go22.uk/rp0271
Age-related decline of progenitor cell activity can be modulated by systemic factors

Human umbilical plasma proteins revitalize hippocampal function in aged mice
Nature – https://go22.uk/rp0272
Human cord plasma revitalizes the hippocampus and improves cognitive function in aged mice

COST: ●●●○○   EASE: ●●●○○   IMPACT: ●●●○○

Commuting

For most people, commuting is an unavoidable part of the work day. The average journey to work lasts fifty-six minutes in the UK. Londoners face the longest commute, averaging seventy-nine minutes, which is longer than the average commute time in any US city.

Longer commute times are associated with raised blood pressure and higher BMI. These are primarily caused by enforced inactivity, and other contributing factors are increased stress and the availability of unhealthy and fast food along transport routes.

The ideal solution is to make your commute physically active. Cycling to work has been shown to reduce the risk of death from cancer and heart disease. It also results in reduced stress through-out the work day.

If your workplace is too far away to walk or cycle to, then consider whether at least part of the journey could be done under your own power. The worst scenario is driving to work because you are sat down door to door. Most journeys that use public transport involve at least some walking, and although people enjoy the freedom of using their own car, concentrating in heavy traffic can be very stressful.

If cycling or walking are not possible, try performing some discrete exercises during your commute. These can be done while standing or sitting. Alternatively, keep moving by walking around while waiting for your bus or train. Short periods of activity can help in the fight against the worse aspects of commuting.

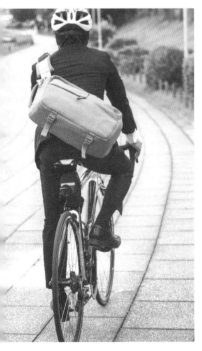

▷ If possible, walk or cycle to work (or part of the journey)

▷ Perform some discrete exercises during your commute

▷ Avoid the temptation of fast food outlets along the way

Tip #96

Information

Health in a Hurry: The impact of commuting
RSPH - https://go22.uk/healthhurry

Commuting: "The Stress That Doesn't Pay"
Psychology Today - https://go22.uk/stresspay

5 Exercises For Your Morning Commute
Alicia Jones - https://go22.uk/5commex

Products

23 of the best commuting bikes
road.cc - https://go22.uk/23bikes
Hybrids, tourers, folders and more

Association between active commuting and incident cardiovascular disease, cancer, mortality
BMJ - https://go22.uk/rp0411
Cycle commuting was associated with a lower risk of CVD, cancer, and all cause mortality

Impact of changes in mode of travel to work on changes in body mass index
Journal of Epidemiology and Community Health - https://go22.uk/rp0412
Switching to more active modes of travel could contribute to reducing population mean BMI

COST: ● ● ● ● ○   EASE: ● ● ● ● ○   IMPACT: ● ● ● ● ○

Lack of control

The next tip examines the health impact of long working hours, however, and perhaps surprisingly, long hours are not the worst factor at work that affects lifespan. Several large-scale reports have all concluded that lack of control at work has the biggest impact on health. This can increase someone's mortality rate (i.e. the chance of dying each year) by 68%. Similarly, lack of job security and heavy demands at work have a bigger impact on mortality than simply working long hours.

Lack of control means having little discretion over, or foresight of, workload and how it is carried out. To cope with the demanding nature of a job it's possible that some employees take up bad habits such as smoking, eating or drinking excessively.

Enlightened companies attempt to craft jobs into something more meaningful to their employees. This not only creates a happier workforce but a more productive one. Of course, not all employers can offer this level of freedom, for example in many engineering jobs there's only one right way to do things.

Tip #97

▶ Don't remain passive – take control at work whenever you can

▶ Accept the things you can't change

▶ If your job is affecting your health then try to find another one

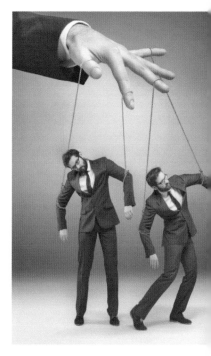

Information
The Tell Tale Signs of Burnout ... Do You Have Them?
Psychology Today - https://go22.uk/burnout

Lack Of Support At Work
Stay Sane At Work - https://go22.uk/sanework

Products
Monster - https://go22.uk/monster
One of the more visited employment websites in the world

Work stress and risk of death in men and women with and without cardiometabolic disease
The Lancet - https://go22.uk/rp0301
Men who experienced job strain had a 68% greater risk of premature death

Workplace stressors & health outcomes: Health policy for the workplace
Behavioural Science & Policy - https://go22.uk/rp0302
44% increase in odds of mortality for people who have low job control

COST: ● ● ○ ○ ○   EASE: ● ● ● ● ○   IMPACT: ● ● ● ○ ○

Long working hours

Long working hours have been linked to many afflictions, such as heart disease, diabetes, depression, anxiety, and poor sleep. Being seen to work late is part of the culture in some countries. Japan has some of the longest working hours in the developed world and even has a term "Karoshi" to describe death attributed to overwork. In Europe, the EU Working Time Directive ensures that employees cannot be made to work more than forty-eight hours per week, and this correlates well with research into working hours and health.

Working over forty hours a week increases the chance of a stroke by 10%, and this jumps to 33% for those working more than fifty-five hours a week. However, a Danish study that followed 150,000 employees for up to fifteen years found a 20% reduction in mortality in those working 41-48 hours per week compared to those working fewer hours (32-40) per week. Although the ideal number of working hours, from a health perspective, is not clear, it seems that working more than forty-eight hours per week starts to have a significant negative impact on health.

As well as avoiding working excessive hours, it is also important to limit the number of weeks worked each year. Another study monitored men at high risk of heart disease and found that the more holidays they took the longer they survived.

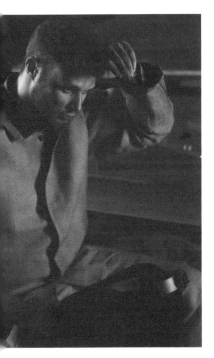

▶ Don't work more than forty-eight hours per week
▶ Take at least two weeks holiday per year
▶ Don't check emails when not at work

Tip #98

Information
Working Long Hours Can Kill You
Inc.com - https://go22.uk/workkills

Long working hours 'health risk'
BBC News - https://go22.uk/longrisk

Rights at work - including working hours, holiday pay and sick pay
Citizens Advice - https://go22.uk/rightsatwork

The association between long working hours and health: A systematic review
Scandinavian Journal of Work, Environment & Health - https://go22.uk/rp0311
Long working hours had significant adverse effects on most health outcomes

Are vacations good for your health? The 9-year mortality experience
Psychosomatic Medicine - https://go22.uk/rp0312
Frequency of annual vacations is associated with a reduced risk of all-cause mortality

COST: ● ● ● ● ●   EASE: ● ● ● ● ○   IMPACT: ● ● ○ ○ ○

Occupation

The number of deaths in the workplace has decreased in recent decades, though there are still over a hundred fatal injuries to workers, every year, in the UK (over 4,000 in the US). The industry with the highest number of deaths is construction, and the most common cause of workplace fatality is a fall from height.

However, the fatal work injury rate gives a better indication of the risk of an individual worker dying on the job. This figure is calculated per 100,000 full-time workers. In the UK the fatal work injury rate is less than two in the construction industry, jumping to eight in agriculture. The industry with the worst rate is waste and recycling, with a rate of ten - equivalent to one death per year per 10,000 workers. Where you work is also a factor – the average fatal work injury rate is eight times higher in the US than in the UK. Older workers also face a higher risk – with 3-5 times the average fatality rate.

However, the rate of deaths due to exposure to harmful substances (occupational health) are far higher than those due to accidents. The Health and Safety Executive estimates that the UK sees around 13,000 deaths each year caused by past exposures, mostly due to lung disease. Due to the long latency between exposure and disease (i.e. current deaths reflect the effect of past working conditions) hopefully these figures do not reflect the risks today. But breathing in dust, gases, fumes and vapours in the workplace can still cause serious lung damage, so you and your employer must control exposure to these substances.

Tip #99

▶ **Work in an industry with a low fatal work injury rate**
▶ **Follow health and safety instructions**
▶ **Take extra care at work as you get older**

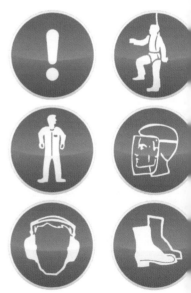

Information

Top 10 Most Dangerous Jobs of 2018
EHS Today - https://go22.uk/top10jobs
Looks at fatal work injury rate (per 100,000 full-time workers) rather than total numbers

Your health, your safety - A brief guide for workers
Health and Safety Executive - https://go22.uk/hseguide

Occupational disease web community
Health and Safety Executive - https://go22.uk/occdisease

Workplace fatal injuries in Great Britain 2018
Health and Safety Executive - https://go22.uk/rp1131
Average annual number of workers killed at work over last five years is 142

Work-related ill health and occupational disease in Great Britain
Health and Safety Executive - https://go22.uk/rp1132
13,000 deaths each year linked to past exposure at work, primarily to chemicals or dust

COST: ● ● ○ ○ ○   EASE: ● ● ○ ○ ○   IMPACT: ● ● ● ○ ○

Cryonics

Unfortunately, many people who are already in their final years are unlikely to survive until the first radical anti-ageing treatments arrive. What if science could give them a second chance? Cryonics is the process of freezing bodies in the hope that future science will advance enough to bring these people back to life. It provides a bridge between today's technology and tomorrow's.

Cryonics is based on the fact that memories and personality are determined by the chemistry and structure of the brain, so if the brain can be preserved then these can be recovered. The process can start as soon as the patient has been declared legally dead. First off, a quick-response team pack the body in ice and inject it with anticoagulants, then blood flow is reinitiated to supply oxygen to the brain during transportation to the cryonics facility. At the facility, the body's fluids are replaced with a cryoprotectant solution to stop harmful ice crystals forming and the body is preserved in liquid nitrogen at -196 °C (-320 °F).

Recovery technology does not yet exist. However, with exponential improvements in medical technology, it is certain that one day the process will be possible. The big question today is whether the current freezing process is precise enough to enable a full recovery at a later date. If too much damage is done during cooling or storage, then there may not be enough information remaining to perform a full restoration, however good recovery technology eventually becomes.

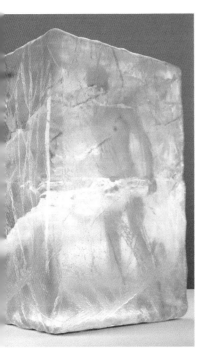

▷ Sign up to have your body preserved with a cryonics company
▷ Consider a head-only service to save money – bodies will be built or grown in the future

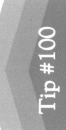

Tip #100

Information
I freeze people to cheat death
BBC Future - https://go22.uk/freezepeople

Organisations
Alcor - https://go22.uk/alcor
Whole body cryopreservation = US$ 200,000
Neurocryopreservation (head only) = US$ 80,000

Cryonics - https://go22.uk/cryonicsorg
Whole body cryopreservation = US$ 28,000

KrioRus - https://go22.uk/kriorus
Whole body/head only = US$ 38,000/16,000

The arrest of biological time as a bridge to engineered negligible senescence
New York Academy of Sciences - https://go22.uk/rp0721
Dogs and cats recovered excellent brain function after 16-60 min of complete cerebral ischemia

Whole body protection during three hours of total circulatory arrest: an experimental study
Cryobiology - https://go22.uk/rp0722
Profound hypothermic conditions was explored in 19 adult mongrel dogs

COST: EASE: IMPACT: ●

Mind uploading

Unlike cryonics (see previous tip) that aims to preserve the mind in its biological brain, mind uploading would allow one's consciousness to be moved to a digital medium. This would provide a more reliable platform where consciousness could more easily be kept safe forever. Here, the problem of storing the brain without damage is replaced with the difficulty of copying the physical structure with sufficient detail to make an accurate facsimile of the mind.

There are thought to be 100 billion neurons in a human brain, each connected to around 7,000 other neurons via 150 trillion synapses, and each firing around 5-50 times every second. This processing power is still beyond the capability of the latest supercomputers but, given the continuation of Moore's Law, it's likely to be possible within the next decade. Significant progress has already been made. The Human Brain Project (one of the EU's largest scientific projects ever) employs 500 scientists to work on the replication of brain architecture and activity on computers.

The big question, also known as the hard problem of consciousness, is whether having made a mathematically exact replica of a brain, which performs in exactly the same way as the original, is it conscious, or is it merely a collection of electronic signals? But maybe that's what consciousness is anyway?

Some companies have already started to make virtual reproductions of the mind, based on a person's emails and online activity. Until full brain simulation is available, this is the only way of ensuring a representation of yourself survives for posterity.

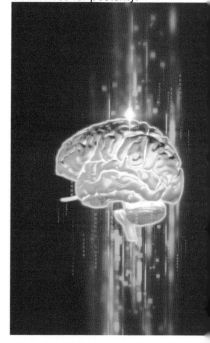

Tip #101

▷ Simulate a mind upload with a virtual reproduction

▷ Record your life digitally to feed into a future AI version of yourself

Information
Digital immortality: a version of you could live forever
MIT Tech Review - https://go22.uk/mitimmortal

Organisations
Terasem Movement - https://go22.uk/terasem
Preserving and downloading human consciousness

2045 Initiative - https://go22.uk/2045init
Transfering personality to a non-biological carrier

Products
Eternime - https://go22.uk/eternime
Oben – https://go22.uk/obenpai

Extremely Scalable Spiking Neuronal Network Simulation Code
Frontiers in Neuroinformatics - https://go22.uk/rp0731
Simulations scale to 10% of human cortex at a resolution of individual neurons & synapses

Reconstruction and Simulation of Neocortical Microcircuitry
Cell - https://go22.uk/rp0732
A neocortical volume of 0.29 ± 0.01 mm3 contains 31,000 neurons

IMAGE ACKNOWLEDGEMENTS

Following images licensed from stock.adobe.com:
Cover illustration silver infinity symbol - valdis torms.
Chapters: Ageing v life extension - eve*, Naked mole rat - belizar, Space colonisation - dottedyeti, How DNA codes - zvitaliy79, Telomeres - designua, The wrapping of DNA - zvitaliy79, How mitochondria convert fuel - Normaals, Tumours are formed - designua, Faulty cells that fail - designua*, Stem cells - metamorworks, Lysosomes - gritsalak, Breaking crosslinks - Ella, Continual rejuvenation - Denis Tabler + Simon, Micro SD - Roman Ivaschenko, Exoskeletons - Chudakov, Molecular nanobots - I.M.R, Robot surgeon - ekkasit919
Tips: #1 BillionPhotos.com, #2 Paul Rookes, #3 springtime78, #5 Gstudio Group, #6 okkijan2010, #7 stuartbur, #8 Monika Wisniewska, #9 Rawpixel.com, #10 patnowa, #11 Tobias Arhelger, #12 Colin & Linda McKie, #13 panptys, #14 alexshyripa, #15 creative soul, #16 Jag_cz, #17 Mara Zemgaliete, #18 exclusive-design, #19 violetkaipa, #20 Jiri Hera, #21 valentinamaslova, #22 creative soul, #23 Harold, #24 Degimages, #25 samuel, #26 marilyn barbone, #27 freshidea, #28 Artistic Endeavor, #29 Bertold Werkmann, #30 bruno135_406, #31 bjphotographs, #32 Francesco Scatena, #33 travelview, #34 Poprotskiy Alexey, #35 WavebreakMediaMicro, #36 Tono Balaguer, #37 Daxiao Productions, #38 pressmaster, #39 molotok289, #40 rastlily, #41 michiel, #42 OlegDoroshin, #43 Nomad_Soul, #44 wirojsid, #45 olly, #46 storm, #47 Vadim Ponomarenko, #48 justtscott, #49 Dmitry, #50 auremar, #51 DragonImages, #52 VadimGuzhva, #53 Anastasiia23, #54 kmiragaya, #55 iceteastock, #56 vectorfusionart, #57 vladi59, #58 JohnKwan, #59 adimas, #60 Alexander Raths, #61 Axel Kock, #62 designua, #63 Robert, #64 Sherry Young, #65 Dmitri Stalnuhhin, #66 Patryk Kosmider, #67 molekuul.be, #69 molekuul.be, #70 matin, #71 Pixelbliss, #72 suprunvitaly, #73 XtravaganT, #74 ImagePixel, #75 zelimirzarkovic, #76 vchalup, #77 VPales, #78 macrovector, #80 Kzenon, #81 StockPhotoPro, #82 Africa Studio, #83 Mikalai Bachkou, #84 Monique, #86 129967211, #87 edwardolive, #88 Andrey Popov, #89 Sherry Young, #90 alexstepanov, #91 molekuul.be, #93 roger ashford, #94 anamejia18, #95 once13, #96 Monet, #97 konradbak, #98 LIGHTFIELD STUDIOS, #99 Onidji, #100 archy13, #101 monsitj

Other sources:
Wright Flyer - Library of Congress, IBM 350 RAMAC - vnunet.com, Outrunning death - CartoonStock (Kim Wark), David H. Murdock - Jim Wezzer, Jeff Bezos - U.S. Department of Defense, Larry Ellison - Oracle Corporate Communications, Peter Thiel - Dan Taylor / Heisenberg Media, Sergey Brin - Steve Jurvetson, Vitalik Buterin - Romanpoet, Phosphatidylcholine - Swanson, Cryotherapy - RudolfSimon, Senescent cells - NIEHS (NIH)

*modified by Adrian Cull

All other images original creations by Adrian Cull.

DATA ATTRIBUTION
UK life expectancy at birth - Office for National Statistics
Your chance of dying doubles every 8 years - Office for National Statistics
Cost of DNA sequencing - www.genome.gov/sequencingcostsdata

Other books you may be interested in

To discover more about futurist thinking and how society is facing radical changes because of changes in technology, as well as people living longer, why not try some of these leading books.

The Singularity Is Near - Ray Kurzweil - https://go22.uk/singisnear
Examines the next step in the evolutionary process of the union of human and machine.

Transcend - Ray Kurzweil – https://go22.uk/transcend
This easy-to-follow program will help you transcend the boundaries of your genetic legacy and live long enough to live forever.

How To Create A Mind - Ray Kurzweil - https://go22.uk/createamind
Explores the limitless potential of reverse-engineering the human brain.

Ending Aging - Aubrey de Grey - https://go22.uk/endingaging
Explains that the aging of the human body, just like the aging of man-made machines, results from an accumulation of various types of damage.

How Not To Die - Michael Greger & Gene Stone - https://go22.uk/hownottodie
Discover the foods scientifically proven to prevent and reverse disease.

Juvenescence: Investing in the age of longevity - Jim Mellon - https://go22.uk/juvenescence
It investigates the new technologies and explains how to benefit from the life extending technologies both personally and professionally.

Abundance - Peter Diamandis - https://go22.uk/abundancepd
We will soon be able to meet and exceed the basic needs of every man, woman and child on the planet. Abundance for all is within our grasp.

Physics of the Future: How Science Will Shape Human Destiny - Michio Kaku - https://go22.uk/physicsfuture
Revolutionary developments in medicine, computers, quantum physics, and space travel that will forever change our way of life and alter the course of civilization itself.

Superintelligence: Paths, Dangers, Strategies - Nick Bostrom - https://go22.uk/superintnb
If machine brains one day come to surpass human brains in general intelligence, then this new superintelligence could become very powerful.

The Knowledge - Lewis Dartnell - https://go22.uk/knowledge
How to rebuild our world from scratch.

ABOUT THE AUTHOR

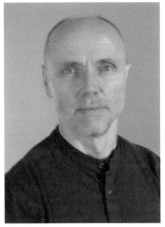

I can only apologise for being the stereotypical white, middle-aged male that seem overly represented in the life extension community. I had no say in my race and gender, but I think I know what influences people, including myself, to become interested in longevity in their forties. Basically, the body starts falling apart! My first experience of this was suffering from frozen shoulder – a painfully stiff shoulder that took almost two years to recover from. There's no genetic or lifestyle reason for getting a frozen shoulder, you're just more likely to get it if you're aged between 40 and 60. Oh. Then my eyes started failing. Classic presbyopia where you can't focus close up because the eye lenses get less flexible with age. I saw a pattern emerging.

Around that time, I read Ray Kurzweil's "The Singularity is Near" and studied with interest the many charts proving the past exponential growth in technology, and what that means for the first half of this century. As medicine has merged with computing, it has entered the information technology age and will now experience the same rapid changes and improvements that we've seen in computers and mobile phones.

I was converted. So, I started collecting articles about anti-ageing research, ways of augmenting the human body and new medical technology, collating them onto my website that eventually became the Live Forever Club. I'm passionate about raising awareness in the general public about the coming revolution in life extension treatments and striving for "equality in longevity" – the club's motto.

Keep up to date with the latest life extension news online with the

Live Forever Club – website (https://liveforever.club), Facebook and Twitter

Printed in Great Britain
by Amazon